Haematology at a Glance

Atul B. Mehta

MA, MD, FRCP, FRCPath
Royal Free and University College School of Medicine
Royal Free Hospital
London

A. Victor Hoffbrand

MA, DM, FRCP, FRCPath, FRCP (Edin), DSc, FMedSci
Royal Free and University College School of Medicine
Royal Free Hospital
London

Fourth edition

WILEY Blackwell

Library of congress cataloging-in-publication data
Mehta, Atul B., author.
    Haematology at a glance / Atul B. Mehta, A. Victor Hoffbrand. – Fourth edition.
       p. ; cm.
Includes bibliographical references and index.
ISBN 978-1-119-96922-8 (pbk. : alk. paper) – ISBN 978-1-118-26119-4 (Mobi) – ISBN 978-1-118-26120-0 (ePdf) – ISBN 978-1-118-26121-7 (ePub) – ISBN 978-1-118-73465-0 – ISBN 978-1-118-73467-4
I. Hoffbrand, A. V., author. II. Title.
[DNLM: 1. Hematologic Diseases. 2. Blood Cells–physiology. 3. Hematopoiesis–physiology. 4. Hemostasis–physiology. WH 120]
RB145
616.1′5–dc23
                            2013018140

A catalogue record for this book is available from the British Library.

Wiley also publishes its books in a variety of electronic formats. Some content that appears in print may not be available in electronic books.

Cover image: © Steve Gschmeissner / Science Photo Library
Cover design by Meaden Creative

Set in 9/11.5 pt Times by Toppan Best-set Premedia Limited
Printed in Singapore by Ho Printing Singapore Pte Ltd

1   2014

Contents

Preface to the fourth edition

Major advances in classification, diagnostic techniques and treatment have occurred over the 4 years since the third edition of this book was published. Much of this new knowledge has depended on the application of molecular techniques for diagnosis and determining treatment and prognosis, particularly for the malignant haematological diseases. New drugs are now available, not only for these diseases but also for treatment of red cell, platelet, thrombotic and bleeding disorders. In order to keep the book to the *at a Glance* size and format, we have included only the new information which represents major change in haematological practice and omitted more detailed knowledge, appropriate for a postgraduate text. The number of diagrams and tables has been increased to make the new information readily accessible to the undergraduate student but overall size of the book has not increased thanks to omission of all obsolete material.

Images have been reproduced, with permission, from Hoffbrand AV, Pettit JE & Vyas P (2010) *Color Atlas of Clinical Hematology*, 4e. Elsevier; Hoffbrand AV & Moss PAH (2011) *Essential Haematology*, 6e Blackwell Publishing Ltd; Hoffbrand AV, Catovsky D, Tuddenham EGD, Green AR *Postgradaute Haematology*, 6e, Blackwell Publishing Ltd, 2011.

We are grateful to June Elliott for her expertise in typing the manuscript, our publishers Wiley Blackwell, and particularly Karen Moore and Rebecca Huxley, for their encouragement and support, and Jane Fallows for the artwork.

Atul B. Mehta
A. Victor Hoffbrand
December 2013

Preface to the first edition

With the ever-increasing complexity of the medical undergraduate curriculum, we feel that there is a need for a concise introduction to clinical and laboratory haematology for medical students. The *at a Glance* format has allowed us to divide the subject into easily digestible slices or bytes of information.

We have tried to emphasize the importance of basic scientific and clinical mechanisms, and common diseases as opposed to rare syndromes. The clinical features and laboratory findings are summarized and illustrated; treatment is briefly outlined.

This book is intended for medical students, but will be useful to anyone who needs a concise and up-to-date introduction to haematology, for example nurses, medical laboratory scientists and those in professions supplementary to medicine.

We particularly thank June Elliott, who has patiently word-processed the manuscript through many revisions, and Jonathan Rowley and his colleagues at Blackwell Science.

Atul B. Mehta
A. Victor Hoffbrand
January 2000

Glossary

Anaemia: a haemoglobin concentration in peripheral blood below normal range for sex and age.

Anisocytosis: variation in size of peripheral blood red cells.

Basophil: a mature circulating white cell with dark purple-staining cytoplasmic granules which may obscure the nucleus.

Chromatin: nuclear material containing DNA and protein.

Clone: a group of cells all derived by mitotic division from a single somatic cell.

CT: computerized scanning.

DIC: disseminated intravascular coagulation.

Eosinophil: mature circulating white cell with multiple orange-staining cytoplasmic granules and two or three nuclear lobes.

Fluorescent *in situ* hybridization (FISH): the use of fluorescently labelled DNA probes which hybridize to chromosomes or sub-chromosomal sequences to detect chromosome deletions or translocations.

Haematocrit: the proportion of a sample of blood taken up by red cells.

Haemoglobin: the red protein in red cells which is composed of four globin chains each containing an iron-containing haem group.

Karyotype: the chromosomal make-up of a cell.

Leucocytosis: a rise in white cell levels in the peripheral blood to above the normal range.

Leucopenia: a fall in white cell (leucocyte) levels in the peripheral blood to below the normal range.

Lymphocyte: a white cell with a single, usually round, nucleus and scanty dark blue-staining cytoplasm. Lymphocytes divide into two main groups: B cells, which produce immunoglobulins; and T cells, which are involved in graft rejection and immunity against viruses.

Macrocytic: red cells of average volume (MCV) above normal.

Mean cell volume (MCV): the average volume of circulating red cells.

Mean corpuscular haemoglobin (MCH): the average haemoglobin content of red blood cells.

Megaloblastic: an abnormal appearance of nucleated red cells in which the nuclear chromatin remains open and fine despite maturation of the cytoplasm.

Microcytic: red cells of average volume (MCV) below normal.

Monocyte: mature circulating white cell with a few pink- or blue-staining cytoplasmic granules, pale blue cytoplasm and a single nucleus. There are usually cytoplasmic vacuoles. In the tissues, the monocyte becomes a macrophage.

MRI: magnetic resonance imaging.

Myeloblast: an early granulocyte precursor containing nucleoli and with a primitive nucleus; there may be some cytoplasmic granules.

Myelocyte: a later granulocyte precursor containing granules, a single lobed nucleus and semi-condensed chromatin.

Neutrophil: a mature white cell containing two to five nuclear lobes and many, fine, reddish or purple cytoplasmic granules.

Normoblast: (erythroblast): nucleated red cell precursor normally found only in bone marrow.

Pancytopenia: a fall in peripheral blood red cell, neutrophil and platelet levels to below normal.

Pappenheimer body: an iron granule in red cells stained by standard (Romanovsky) stain.

Paraprotein: a γ-globulin band on protein electrophoresis consisting of identical molecules derived from a clone of plasma cells.

PET scan: positron emission tomography scan used to detect the sites of active disease, e.g. lymphoma.

Phagocyte: a white blood cell that engulfs bacteria or dead tissue. It includes neutrophils and monocytes (macrophages).

Plasma cell: usually an oval-shaped cell, derived from a B lymphocyte, which secretes immunoglobulin. Plasma cells are found in normal bone marrow but not in normal peripheral blood.

Platelet: the smallest cell in peripheral blood, it is non-nucleated and involved in promoting haemostasis.

Poikilocytosis: variation in shape of peripheral blood red cells.

Polycythaemia: a haemoglobin concentration in peripheral blood above normal range for age and sex.

Red cell: mature non-nucleated cell carrying haemoglobin. The most abundant cell in peripheral blood.

Reticulocyte: a non-nucleated young red cell still containing RNA and found in peripheral blood.

Sideroblast: a nucleated red cell precursor found in marrow and containing iron granules, which appear blue with Perls' stain.

Siderocyte: a mature red cell containing iron granules and found in peripheral blood or marrow.

Stem cell: resides in the bone marrow and by division and differentiation gives rise to all the blood cells. The stem cell also reproduces itself. Some stem cells circulate in the peripheral blood.

Thrombocytopenia: a platelet level in peripheral blood below the normal range.

Thrombocytosis: a platelet level in peripheral blood above the normal range.

Tissue factor: a protein on the surface of cells which initiates blood coagulation.

White cell (leucocyte): nucleated cell that circulates in peripheral blood and whose main function is combating infections. White cells include granulocytes (neutrophils, eosinophils, and basophils), monocytes and lymphocytes.

von Willebrand factor: a plasma protein that carries factor VIII and mediates the adhesion of platelets to the vessel wall.

Normal values

Normal peripheral blood count

Cell	Normal concentration
Haemoglobin	115–155 g/L (female)
	135–175 g/L (male)
Red cell	$3.9–5.6 \times 10^{12}$/L (female)
	$4.5–6.5 \times 10^{12}$/L (male)
Reticulocyte	0.5–3.5%
	$\sim25–95 \times 10^{9}$/L
White cells	$4.0–11.0 \times 10^{9}$/L
Neutrophils	$1.8–7.5 \times 10^{3}$/L
	$(1.5–7.5 \times 10^{9}$/L in black people)
Eosinophils	$0.04–0.4 \times 10^{9}$/L
Basophils	$0.01–0.1 \times 10^{9}$/L
Monocytes	$0.2–0.8 \times 10^{9}$/L
Lymphocytes	$1.5–3.0 \times 10^{9}$/L
Haematocrit	0.38–0.54
Mean cell volume	80–100 (Fig. 8.2)
Mean cell haemoglobin	27–33 (Fig. 8.2)
Haematinics	
Serum iron	10–30 µmol/L
Total iron binding capacity	40–75 µmol/L (2–4 g/L as transferrin)
Serum ferritin	40–340 µg/L (males)
	15–150 µg/L (females)
Serum folate	3.0–15.0 µg/L (4–30 nmol/L)
Red cell folate	160–640 µg/L (360–1460 nmol/L)
Serum vitamin B_{12}	160–925 µg/L (120–682 pmol/L)

About the companion website

Visit the companion website at:

www.ataglanceseries.com/haematology

The website includes:

• Multiple-Choice Questions

• Case studies from the book

All of these are interactive so that you can easily test yourself on the topics in each chapter.

Scan this QR code to visit the companion website.

Haemopoiesis: physiology and pathology

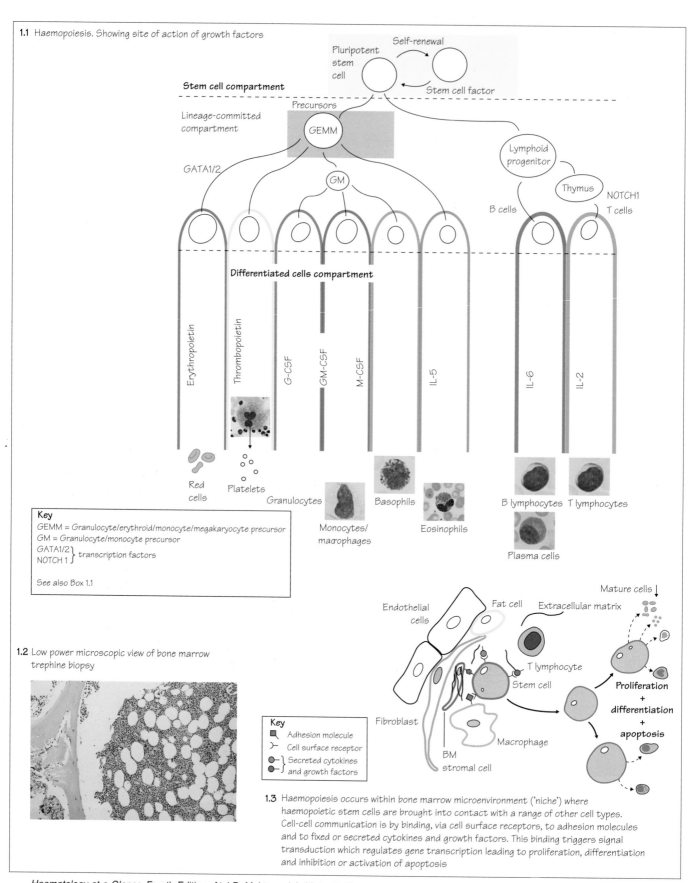

1.1 Haemopoiesis. Showing site of action of growth factors

Key

GEMM = Granulocyte/erythroid/monocyte/megakaryocyte precursor
GM = Granulocyte/monocyte precursor
GATA1/2 } transcription factors
NOTCH 1 }

See also Box 1.1

1.2 Low power microscopic view of bone marrow trephine biopsy

Key

▪ Adhesion molecule
⌐ Cell surface receptor
● } Secreted cytokines
● } and growth factors

1.3 Haemopoiesis occurs within bone marrow microenvironment ('niche') where haemopoietic stem cells are brought into contact with a range of other cell types. Cell-cell communication is by binding, via cell surface receptors, to adhesion molecules and to fixed or secreted cytokines and growth factors. This binding triggers signal transduction which regulates gene transcription leading to proliferation, differentiation and inhibition or activation of apoptosis

Haematology at a Glance, Fourth Edition. Atul B. Mehta and A. Victor Hoffbrand.

1.4 The signal transduction pathway. This is a series of biochemical pathways whereby a message from the cell surface can be transmitted to the nucleus (see pg 12)

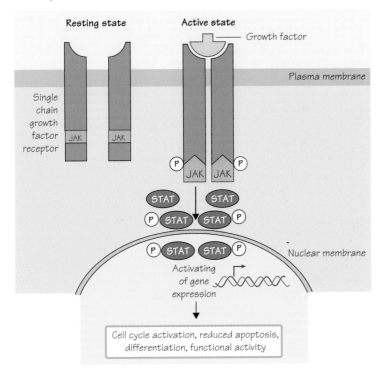

1.5 Apoptosis. Activation of caspases by DNA damage, release of cytochrome C from mitochondria and by FAS ligand. Apoptosis is inhibited by BCL-2

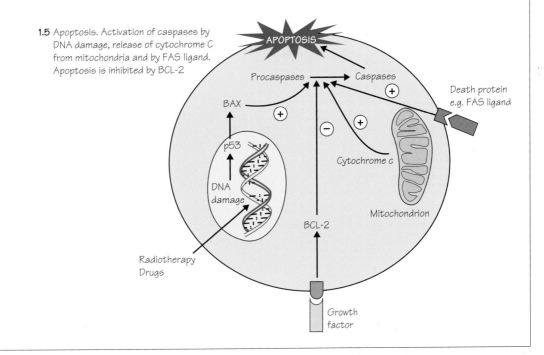

Definition and sites

Haemopoiesis is the process whereby blood cells are made (Fig. 1.1). The yolk sac, and later the liver and spleen, are important in fetal life, but after birth normal haemopoiesis is restricted to the bone marrow.

Infants have haemopoietic marrow in all bones, but in adults it is in the central skeleton and proximal ends of long bones (normal fat to haemopoietic tissue ratio of about 50:50) (Fig. 1.2). Expansion of haemopoiesis down the long bones may occur in bone marrow malignancy, e.g. in leukaemias, or when there is increased demand, e.g. chronic haemolytic anaemias. The liver and spleen can resume extramedullary haemopoiesis when there is marrow replacement, e.g. in myelofibrosis, or excessive demand, e.g. in severe haemolytic anaemias such as thalassaemia major.

Stem and progenitor cells

Haemopoiesis involves the complex physiological processes of proliferation, differentiation and apoptosis (programmed cell death). The bone marrow produces more than a million red cells per second in addition to similar numbers of white cells and platelets. This capacity can be increased in response to increased demand. A common primitive stem cell in the marrow has the capacity to self-replicate and to give rise to increasingly specialized or commited progenitor cells which, after many (13–16) cell divisions within the marrow, form the mature cells (red cells, granulocytes, monocytes, platelets and lymphocytes) of the peripheral blood (Fig. 1.1). The earliest recognizable red cell precursor is a pronormoblast and for granulocytes or monocytes, a myeloblast. An early lineage division is between lymphoid and myeloid cells. Stem and progenitor cells cannot be recognized morphologically; they resemble lymphocytes. Progenitor cells can be detected by *in vitro* assays in which they form colonies (e.g. colony-forming units for granulocytes and monocytes, CFU-GM, or for red cells, BFU-E and CFU-E). Stem and progenitor cells also circulate in the peripheral blood and can be harvested for use in stem cell transplantation.

The stromal cells of the marrow (fibroblasts, endothelial cells, macrophages, fat cells) have adhesion molecules that react with corresponding ligands on the stem cells to maintain their viability and to localize them correctly (Fig. 1.3). With osteoblasts these stromal cells form 'niches' in which stem cells reside. The marrow also contains mesenchymal stem cells that can form cartilage, fibrous tissue, bone and endothelial cells.

Growth factors

Haemopoiesis is regulated by growth factors (GFs) (Box 1.1) which usually act in synergy. These are glycoproteins produced by stromal cells, T lymphocytes, the liver and, for erythropoietin, the kidney (Fig. 2.6). While some GFs act mainly on primitive cells, others act on later cells already committed to a particular lineage. GFs also affect the function of mature cells. The signal is transmitted to the nucleus by a cascade of phosphorylation reactions (Fig. 1.4). GFs inhibit apoptosis (Fig. 1.5) of their target cells. GFs in clinical use include erythropoietin, granulocyte colony-stimulating factor (G-CSF), and analogues of thrombopoietin.

Box 1.1 Haemopoietic growth factors

Act on stromal cells
- IL-1 (stimulate production of GM-CSF, G-CSF, M-CSF, IL-6)
- TNF

  Act on pluripotential cells
- Stem cell factor

  Act on early multipotential cells
- IL-3
- IL-4
- IL-6
- GM-CSF

  Act on committed progenitor cells*
- G-CSF
- M-CSF
- IL-5 (eosinophil CSF)
- Erythropoietin
- Thrombopoietin

G-CSF, granulocyte colony-stimulating factor; GM-CSF, granulocyte-macrophage colony-stimulating factor; IL, interleukin; M-CSF, monocyte colony-stimulating factor; TNF, tumour necrosis factor
*These growth factors (especially G-CSF and thrombopoietin) also act on earlier cells

---

Transcription factors

These proteins regulate expression of genes e.g. GATA1/2 and NOTCH. They bind to specific DNA sequences and contribute to the assembly of a gene transcription complex at the gene promotor.

Signal transduction (Fig. 1.4)

The binding of a GF with its surface receptor on the haemopoietic cell activates by phosphorylation, a complex series of biochemical reactions by which the message is transmitted to the nucleus. Figure 1.4 illustrates a typical pathway in which the signal is transmitted to transcription factors in the nucleus by phosphorylation of JAK2 and STAT molecules. The transcription factors in turn activate or inhibit gene transcription. The signal may activate pathways that cause the cell to enter cell cycle (replicate), differentiate, maintain viability (inhibition of apoptosis) or increase functional activity (e.g. enhancement of bacterial cell killing by neutrophils). Disturbances of these pathways due to acquired genetic changes, e.g. mutations, deletion or translocation, often involving transcription factors, underlie many of the malignant diseases of the bone marrow such as the acute or chronic leukaemias and lymphomas.

Apoptosis

Apoptosis (programmed cell death) is the process by which most cells in the body die. The individual cell is activated so that intracellular proteins (caspases) kill the cell by an active process. Caspases may be activated by external stimuli as intracellular damage, e.g. to DNA (Fig. 1.5).

Assessment of haemopoiesis

Haemopoiesis can be assessed clinically by performing a full blood count (see Normal values). Bone marrow aspiration also allows assessment of the later stages of maturation of haemopoietic cells (Fig. 7.3; see Chapter 7 for indications). Trephine biopsy (Fig. 1.2) provides a core of bone and bone marrow to show architecture. Reticulocytes (see Chapter 2) are young red cells. Assessment of their numbers can be performed by automated cell counters and will give an indication of the output of young red cells by the bone marrow. As a general rule, the action of GFs increases the number of young cells in response to demand.

2 Normal blood cells I: red cells

2.1 Normal blood film

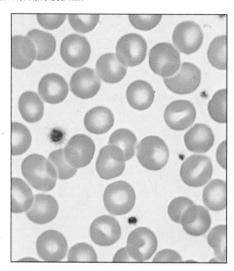

2.2 Normal adult haemoglobin contains four globin (polypeptide) chains (α_1 α_2, β_1, β_2), each with its own haem molecule. These chains undergo conformational change and move with respect to each other when binding O_2 and CO_2. 2,3-Diphosphoglycerate (2,3-DPG) binds between the β chains to reduce affinity for O_2 and allow O_2 release to the tissues

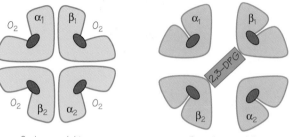

Oxyhaemoglobin

Deoxyhaemoglobin

2.3 The p50 is the partial pressure of oxygen at which haemoglobin is 50% saturated (red curve, normally 27mmHg). Decreased oxygen affinity, with increasing p50 (green curve) occurs as carbon dioxide concentration increases or pH decreases (Bohr effect) or 2,3-DPG levels rise. Increased oxygen affinity occurs during the opposite circumstances or may be a characteristic of a variant haemoglobin, which may lead to polycythaemia (see Chapter 27), e.g. Hb Chesapeake or Hb F

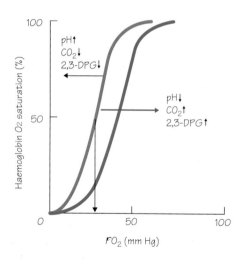

Haematology at a Glance, Fourth Edition. Atul B. Mehta and A. Victor Hoffbrand.

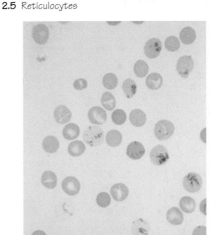

Peripheral blood cells

Normal peripheral blood contains mature cells that do not undergo further division. Their numbers are counted by automatic cell counters which also determine red cell size and haemoglobin content.

Red cells (erythrocytes)

Red cells are the most numerous of the peripheral blood cells (10^{12}/L) (Fig. 2.1). They are among the simplest of cells in vertebrates and are highly specialized for their function, which is to carry oxygen to all parts of the body and to return carbon dioxide to the lungs. Red cells exist only within the circulation – unlike many types of white blood cells they cannot traverse the endothelial membrane. They are larger than the diameter of the capillaries in the microcirculation. This requires them to have a flexible membrane.

Haemoglobin

Red cells contain haemoglobin which allows them to carry oxygen (O_2) and carbon dioxide (CO_2). Haemoglobin is composed of four polypeptide globin chains each with an iron containing haem molecule (Fig. 2.2). Three types of haemoglobin occur in normal adult blood: haemoglobin A, A_2 and F (Table 2.1). The ability of haemoglobin to bind O_2 is measured as the haemoglobin–O_2 dissociation curve. Raised concentrations of 2,3-DPG, H^+ ions or CO_2 decrease O_2 affinity, allowing more O_2 delivery to tissues (Fig. 2.3). Some pathological variant haemoglobins are similar to Hb F in having a higher oxygen affinity than Hb A (Fig. 2.3); this leads, in adults, to a state of relative tissue hypoxia and the body compensates by increasing the number of red cells (secondary

Table 2.1 Normal haemoglobins			
	Hb A	Hb A_2	Hb F
Structure	$\alpha_2\beta_2$	$\alpha_2\delta_2$	$\alpha_2\gamma_2$
Normal adult (%)	96–98	1.5–3.5	0.5–0.8

polycythaemia, see Chapter 26). In contrast, some pathological variant haemoglobins (e.g. Hb S, the major haemoglobin in sickle cell disease, see Chapter 17) have a lower oxygen affinity than Hb A (Fig. 2.3). This allows individuals to maintain a higher than normal tissue oxygenation for a given haemoglobin concentration.

Red cell production

The earliest recognizable red cell precursor is a pronormoblast (Fig. 2.4). This arises from a progenitor cell CFU-E committed to red cell production. The pronormoblast has an open nucleus, a cytoplasm that stains dark blue (because of a high RNA content) with the usual (Romanowsky) stain for bone marrow blood cells. By a series of cell divisions and differentiation (with haemoglobin formation in the cytoplasm), the cells develop through different normoblast stages until they lose their nuclei. Ten to fifteen percent of developing erythroblasts die within the marrow without producing mature red cells. This **'ineffective erythropoiesis'** is increased and becomes an important cause of reduced haemoglobin concentration (anaemia) in various

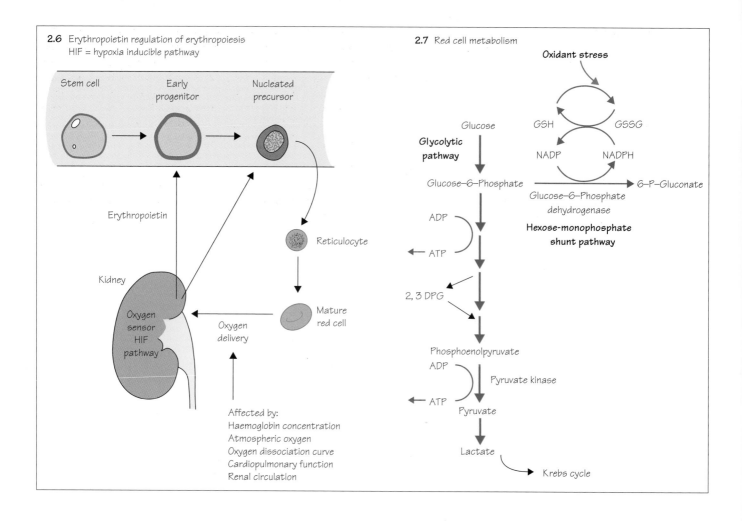

2.6 Erythropoietin regulation of erythropoiesis
HIF = hypoxia inducible pathway

2.7 Red cell metabolism

pathological states, e.g. thalassaemia major, myelofibrosis, myelodysplasia and megaloblastic anaemia.

Reticulocytes

These are newly formed red cells that have lost a nucleus but retain some RNA. They can synthesise proteins. The RNA is lost after about 48 hours and the reticulocytes are then mature red cells. The RNA can be stained with supravital dyes before the cells have been 'fixed' on a blood film. Modern automatic counters are now used to measure reticulocytes in absolute numbers and as a percentage of the total red cells. Reticulocytes can also be counted on a specially stained blood film as a percentage of the red cells (Fig. 2.5). The normal range is 1–3% of red cells or $50 - 150 \times 10^9$/L. The reticulocyte count is a measure of new red cell production by the marrow. It is raised after haemorrhage or haemolysis when extra red cell production is needed. It is low if the marrow is incapable of normal red cell production, e.g. because of malignant infiltration or aplastic anaemia. More common causes include lack of iron, vitamin B_{12} or folate, or a chronic systemic disease or lack of erythropoietin in kidney disease.

Erythropoietin

This hormone controls the production of red cells. It is produced in the peritubular complex of the kidney (90%), liver and other organs (Fig. 2.6). Erythropoietin stimulates mixed lineage and red cell progenitors as well as pronormoblasts and early erythroblasts to proliferate, differentiate and synthesize haemoglobin (Table 2.1). Erythropoietin secretion is stimulated by reduced O_2 supply to the kidney receptor. Thus, the principal stimuli to red cell production are tissue hypoxia and reduced haemoglobin concentration (anaemia) which act through the HIF pathway. Exogenous erythropoietin binds to the erythropoietin receptor on the surface of the red cell and initiates a signal transduction (see Fig. 1.4) by phosphorylation of the Janus kinase 2 (JAK2). This in turn induces gene transcription and red cell proliferation. Mutations in JAK2 underlie pathologically increased red cell production in polycythaemia rubra vera (PRV, see Chapter 27).

Red cell metabolism

Mature red cells have no nucleus, ribosomes or mitochondria. They survive for about 120 days before being removed by macrophages of the reticuloendothelial system (see Chapter 3). Red cells are capable of only the simplest metabolic pathways.

The **glycolytic pathway** (Fig. 2.7) is the main source of energy (ATP) required to maintain red cell shape and deformability. The hexose monophosphate 'shunt' (pentose phosphate) pathway provides the main source of reduced nicotinamide adenine dinucleotide phosphate (NADPH), which maintains reduced glutathione (GSH) and protects haemoglobin and the membrane proteins against oxidant damage (Fig. 2.7). Oxygen radicals are generated by the constant oxygenation and deoxygenation of haemoglobin.

Red cell membrane is a bipolar lipid layer that anchors surface antigens. It has a protein skeleton (spectrin, actin, protein 4.1 and ankyrin) which maintains the red cell's biconcave shape and deformability. These proteins contain several sulphydryl (-SH) groups which are essential for the maintenance of their tertiary structure and therefore the structural integrity of the red cell. These sulphydryl groups require NADPH generated by the pentose phosphate pathway to protect them from oxygen radicals.

Haematinics

Haematinics are naturally occurring substances, absorbed from the diet, that are essential for red cell production. They include minerals (e.g. iron) and vitamins (e.g. B_{12}, B_6 and folate).

Normal blood cells II: granulocytes, monocytes and the reticuloendothelial system

3.1 The reticuloendothelial system. APC, antigen presenting cell

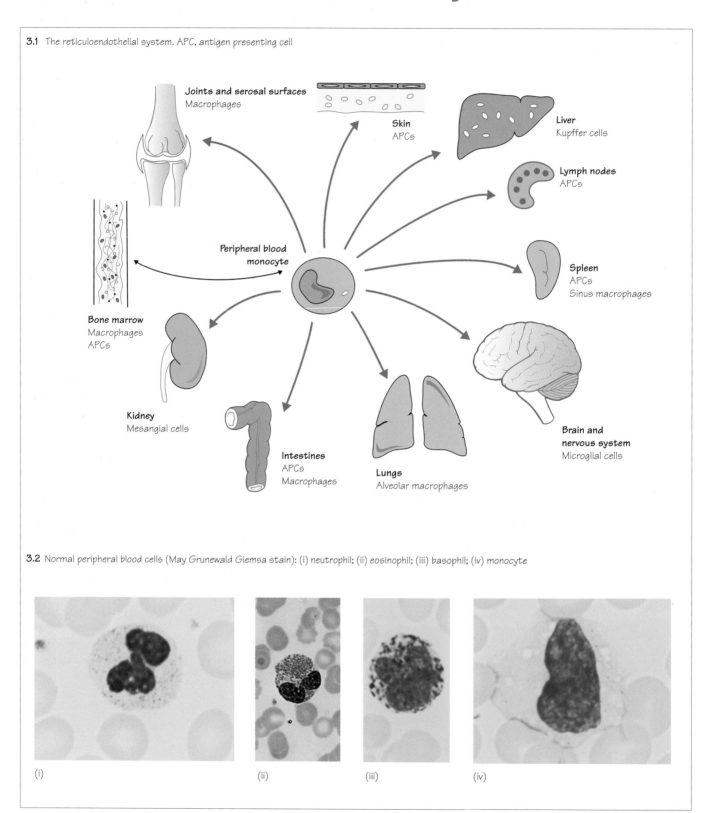

3.2 Normal peripheral blood cells (May Grunewald Giemsa stain): (i) neutrophil; (ii) eosinophil; (iii) basophil; (iv) monocyte

(i)   (ii)   (iii)   (iv)

Haematology at a Glance, Fourth Edition. Atul B. Mehta and A. Victor Hoffbrand.

18 © 2014 John Wiley & Sons, Ltd. Published 2014 by John Wiley & Sons, Ltd. Companion Website: www.ataglanceseries.com/haematology

Normal white blood cells (leucocytes) in peripheral blood are of five types: three of them contain granules and are termed granulocytes (neutrophils or polymorphs, eosinophils and basophils) and the other two types are monocytes and lymphocytes (see Chapter 4). Granulocyte and monocyte production occurs in the bone marrow and is controlled by growth factors (see Table 1.1). External stimuli (e.g. infection, fever, inflammation, allergy and trauma) act on stromal and other cells to liberate cytokines, e.g. interleukin 1 (IL-1) and tumour necrosis factor (TNF), which then stimulate increased production of these growth factors. The earliest recognizable granulocyte precursors are myeloblasts. These undergo a final division followed by further maturation into promyelocytes, myelocytes, metamyelocytes and, finally, mature granulocytes (neutrophils, eosinophils and basophils).

Function of white cells

The primary function of white cells is to protect the body against infection. They work closely with proteins of the immune response, immunoglobulins and complement. Neutrophils, eosinophils, basophils and monocytes are all phagocytes; they ingest and destroy pathogens and cell debris. Phagocytes are attracted to bacteria at the site of inflammation by chemotactic substances released from damaged tissues and by complement components. Opsonization is the coating of cells or foreign particles by immunoglobulin or complement; this aids phagocytosis (engulfment) because phagocytes have immunoglobulin Fc and complement C3b receptors (see below). Killing involves reduction of pH within the phagocytic vacuole, the release of granule contents and the production of antimicrobial oxidants and superoxides (the 'respiratory burst').

Neutrophils

Neutrophils (polymorphs) (Fig. 3.2(i)) are the most numerous peripheral blood leucocytes. They have a short lifespan of approximately 10 hours in the circulation. About 50% of neutrophils in peripheral blood are attached to the walls of blood vessels (marginating pool). Primary neutrophil granules, present from the promyelocyte stage, contain lysosomal enzymes. Secondary granules containing other enzymes (peroxidase, lysosyme, alkaline phosphatase and lactoferrin) appear later. Neutrophils enter tissues by migrating in response to chemotactic factors. Migration, phagocytosis and killing are energy-dependent functions. The concentration of neutrophils in the blood may be lower in certain racial populations, e.g. Afro-Caribbean, Middle Eastern than in Caucasians.

Eosinophils

Eosinophils have similar kinetics of production, differentiation and circulation to neutrophils; the growth factor IL-5 is important in regulating their production. They have a bilobed nucleus (Fig. 3.2(ii)) and red–orange staining granules (containing histamine). They are particularly important in the response to parasitic and allergic diseases. Release of their granule contents onto larger pathogens (e.g. helminths) aids their destruction and subsequent phagocytosis.

Basophils

Basophils are closely related to mast cells (small darkly staining cells in the bone marrow and tissues). Both are derived from granulocyte precursors in the bone marrow. They are the least numerous of peripheral blood leucocytes and have large dark purple granules which may obscure the nucleus (Fig. 3.2(iii)). The granule contents include histamine and heparin and are released following binding of IgE to surface receptors. They play an important part in immediate hypersensitivity reactions. Mast cells also have an important role in defence against allergens and parasitic pathogens.

Monocytes

Monocytes (Fig. 3.2(iv)) circulate for 20–40 hours and then enter tissues, become macrophages, mature and carry out their principal functions. Within tissues, they survive for many days, possibly months. They have variable morphology in peripheral blood, but are mononuclear, have greyish cytoplasm with vacuoles and small granules. Within tissues, they often have long cytoplasmic projections allowing them to communicate widely with other cells.

Reticuloendothelial system

This is used to describe monocyte-derived cells (Fig. 3.1) which are distributed throughout the body in multiple organs and tissues. The system includes Kupffer cells in the liver, alveolar macrophages in the lung, mesangial cells in the kidney, microglial cells in the brain and macrophages within the bone marrow, spleen, lymph nodes, skin and serosal surfaces. The principal functions of the reticuloendothelial system (RES) are to:
• phagocytose and destroy pathogens and cellular debris, e.g. red cell debris;
• process and present antigens to lymphoid cells (the antigen-presenting cells react principally with T cells with whom they 'interdigitate' in lymph nodes, spleen, thymus, bone marrow and tissues);
• produce cytokines (e.g. IL-1) which regulate and participate within cytokine and growth factor networks governing haemopoiesis, inflammation and cellular responses.

The cells of the RES are particularly localized in tissues that may come into contact with external allergens or pathogens. The main organs of the RES allow its cells to communicate with lymphoid cells, and include the liver, spleen, lymph nodes, bone marrow, thymus and intestinal tract (or mucosa-) associated lymphoid tissue.

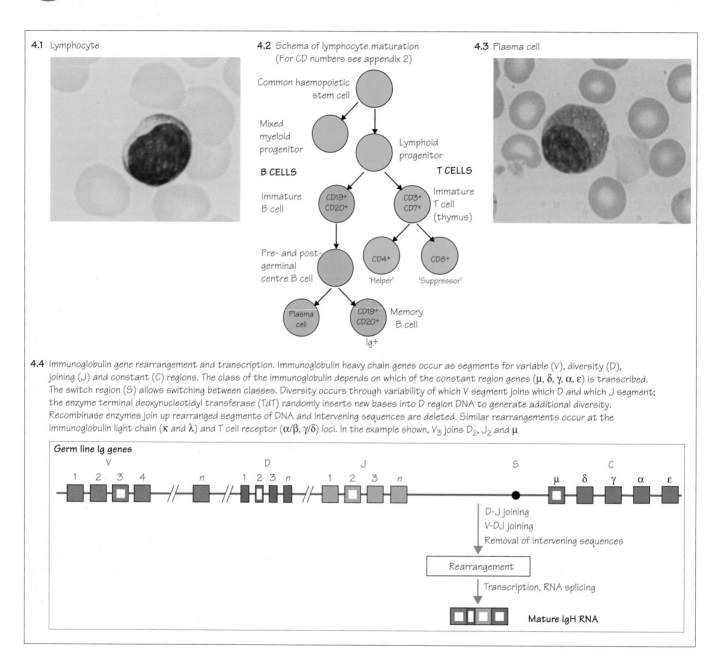

4.1 Lymphocyte

4.2 Schema of lymphocyte maturation
(For CD numbers see appendix 2)

Common haemopoietic stem cell

Mixed myeloid progenitor

Lymphoid progenitor

B CELLS

T CELLS

Immature B cell — CD19+ CD20+

CD3+ CD7+ — Immature T cell (thymus)

CD4+ 'Helper'

CD8+ 'Suppressor'

Pre- and post-germinal centre B cell

Plasma cell

CD19+ CD20+ Ig+ — Memory B cell

4.3 Plasma cell

4.4 Immunoglobulin gene rearrangement and transcription. Immunoglobulin heavy chain genes occur as segments for variable (V), diversity (D), joining (J) and constant (C) regions. The class of the immunoglobulin depends on which of the constant region genes (μ, δ, γ, α, ε) is transcribed. The switch region (S) allows switching between classes. Diversity occurs through variability of which V segment joins which D and which J segment; the enzyme terminal deoxynucleotidyl transferase (TdT) randomly inserts new bases into D region DNA to generate additional diversity. Recombinase enzymes join up rearranged segments of DNA and intervening sequences are deleted. Similar rearrangements occur at the immunoglobulin light chain (κ and λ) and T cell receptor (α/β, γ/δ) loci. In the example shown, V_3 joins D_2, J_2 and μ

Germin line Ig genes

V 1 2 3 4 ... n
D 1 2 3 n
J 1 2 3 n
S
C μ δ γ α ε

D-J joining
V-DJ joining
Removal of intervening sequences

Rearrangement

Transcription, RNA splicing

Mature IgH RNA

Haematology at a Glance, Fourth Edition. Atul B. Mehta and A. Victor Hoffbrand.

Table 4.1 Classification of mature lymphocytes

Class	Function	Proportion in peripheral blood	Phenotype
B cells	Secretion of antibodies	20–40%	CD19$^+$, CD20$^+$
Helper T cells	Release of cytokines and growth factors that regulate other immune cells	30–60%	CD3$^+$, CD4$^+$, TCR αβ
Cytotoxic T cells	Lysis of virally infected cells, tumour cells, non-self cells	10–30%	CD3$^+$, CD8$^+$, TCR αβ
NK cells	Lysis of virally infected and tumour cells	2–10%	CD16$^+$, CD56$^+$, CD3$^-$

Lymphocytes (Fig. 4.1) are an essential component of the immune response and are derived from haemopoietic stem cells. A common lymphoid stem cell gives rise to daughter cells which undergo differentiation and proliferation (Fig. 4.2).

Lymphocyte maturation occurs principally in bone marrow for B cells and in the thymus for T cells, but also involves the lymph nodes, liver, spleen and other parts of the reticuloendothelial system. B cells mediate humoral or antibody-mediated immunity while T cells are responsible for cell-mediated immunity. Lymphocytes can be characterized on the basis of the antigens expressed on the surface of the cell (Table 4.1). These differ according to the lineage and level of maturity of the cell. The cluster of differentiation (CD) nomenclature system has evolved as a means of classifying these antigens according to their reaction with monoclonal antibodies (see Appendix). Lymphocytes have the longest lifespan of any leucocyte, some (e.g. 'memory' B cells) living for many years.

Immune response

The immune response involves a complex interaction of cells (including B lymphocytes, T lymphocytes, macrophages), proteins (immunoglobulins, complement) and lipids (e.g. glycosphingolipids) whereby the body responds to infection, injury and neoplasia. Inflammation is a non-specific outcome of the immune response. Specificity of the immune response derives from amplification of antigen-selected T and B cells. The mature B cells that manufacture immunoglobulin are termed plasma cells (Fig. 4.3). The T-cell receptor (TCR) on T cells and surface membrane immunoglobulin (sIg) on B cells are receptor molecules that have a variable and a constant portion. The variability ensures that a specific antigen is recognized by a lymphocyte with a matching variable receptor region. The genetic mechanisms required to generate the required diversity are common to T and B cells (Fig. 4.4). They involve rearrangement of variable, joining, diversity and constant region genes to generate genes coding for surface receptors (sIg or TCR) capable of reacting specifically with one of an enormous array of antigens.

The generation of a specific immune response usually involves interaction between the antigen and T cells, B cells and antigen-presenting cells (APCs), which are specialised macrophages. Mature T cells are of three main types: helper cells which express the CD4 antigen and generally augment B cell responses; suppressor cells which express CD8 and generally suppress B cells; and cytotoxic cells which also express CD8. Developing T cells are 'educated' in the thymus to react only to foreign antigens, and to develop tolerance to self-human leucocyte antigens (HLA). B cells can also interact directly with antigen. Adhesion molecules mediate these cellular interactions.

Reaction between antigen and appropriate receptor (sIg or TCR) leads to B or T cellular proliferation (clonal selection) and differentiation. Antibody is produced to the antigen and cells presenting the antigen are killed by macrophages or T cells. A key location for clonal selection is the germinal centre of lymph nodes and spleen (Fig. 5.1). 'Pre-germinal centre' B cells are less mature and have not undergone further mutation of nucleotide residues at the heavy chain variable region (VH) gene locus. More mature B cells are 'post-germinal centre' and have mutated VH genes. B-cell malignancies derived from these B cells (e.g. chronic lymphocytic leukaemia, CLL, see Fig. 31.1) will reproduce this feature, and it is noteworthy that the degree of somatic mutation at the IgH immunoglobulin gene locus relates to prognosis of the leukaemia. Malignancies derived from very immature lymphocytes (e.g. B and T cell-derived acute lymphoblastic leukaemia, ALL, see Chapter 22) are generally positive for the enzyme TdT (terminal deoxynucleotidyl transferase) which is responsible for much of the generation of genetic diversity in B or T cells.

Natural killer cells

Natural killer cells are neither T nor B cells, though are often CD8$^+$. They characteristically have prominent granules and are often large granular lymphocytes. These cells are not governed like T and B cells by HLA restriction, and are usually activated by a class of cytokines termed interferons. They can kill target cells by direct adhesion, secretion of their granule contents causing cell lysis.

Immunoglobulins

These are gammaglobulins produced by plasma cells. There are five main groups: IgG, IgM, IgA, IgD and IgE. Each is composed of light and heavy chains, and each chain is made up of variable, joining and constant regions (Fig. 4.4).

Complement

This is a group of plasma proteins and cell surface receptors which, if activated, interact with cellular and humoral elements in the inflammatory response (Fig. 4.5). The complete molecule is capable of direct lysis of cell membranes and of pathogens sensitized by antibody. The C3b component coats cells making them sensitive to phagocytosis by macrophages. C3a and C5a may also activate chemotaxis by phagocytes and activate mast cells and basophils to release mediators of inflammation.

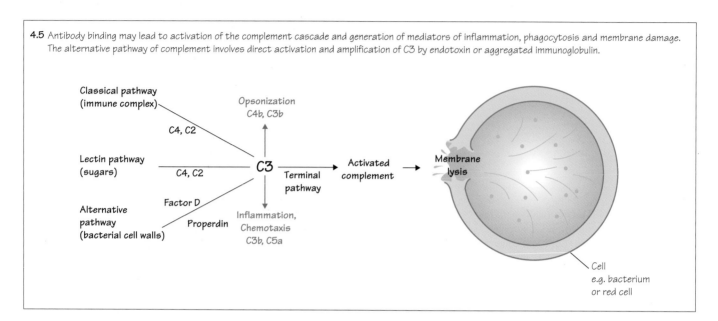

4.5 Antibody binding may lead to activation of the complement cascade and generation of mediators of inflammation, phagocytosis and membrane damage. The alternative pathway of complement involves direct activation and amplification of C3 by endotoxin or aggregated immunoglobulin.

5.1 Diagramatic section through a lymph node. The marginal zone is a thin rim around the mantle. F, follicle with germinal centre; MC, medullary cords; PC, paracortex (interfollicular area); S, sinus.

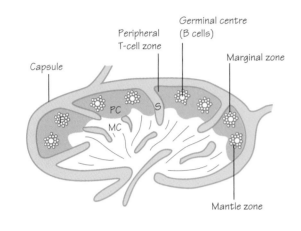

5.2 Diagrammatic section through the spleen. The splenic arterioles are surrounded by a periarteriolar lymphatic sheath – the 'white pulp'. This is composed of T cells and germinal centre B cells. Blood then flows through the meshwork of the red pulp to find its way into sinuses which are the venous outflow. Part of the splenic blood flow bypasses this filtration process to pass directly through to the veins via the splenic cords.

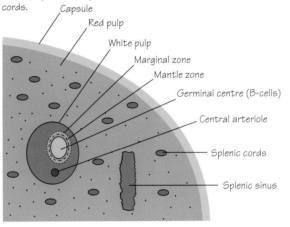

The lymph nodes and spleen are important organs of the body's immune system and reticuloendothelial system (RES). They represent key areas where antigen (processed by the cells of the RES) can be presented by specialized macrophages, antigen-presenting cells, to the cells of the immune system (B and T cells). The anatomy of lymph nodes and spleen are illustrated in Figs 5.1 and 5.2. A common feature is the presence of germinal centres (Fig. 5.1), which are an important location for B-cell maturation and proliferation.

The spleen has a specialized circulatory network which allows it to perform its functions. Red cells are concentrated from the arteriolar circulation and pass through the endothelial meshwork of the red pulp to the sinuses of the venous circulation. This process brings antigens, particulate matter (e.g. opsonized bacteria), effete cells or unwanted material in red cells (e.g. nuclear remnants, iron granules) in proximity with the specialized cells of the RES, the splenic macrophages. These macrophages and lymphocytes occupy the densely cellular areas of the spleen termed the white pulp.

Lymph and the lymphatic system

Lymph is a fluid that is derived from blood as a filtrate and circulates around the body (including lymph nodes, liver, spleen and serosal surfaces) in lymph vessels (the lymphatic system). Lymph is rich in lymphocytes, which are returned to the blood circulation via the azygous vein and thoracic duct which drain lymph into the right atrium. Obstruction of the lymph vessels (e.g. by external compression or as a result of pathology within lymph nodes) leads to swelling (oedema or lymphoedema). Causes of lymph node enlargement are listed in Chapter 19, Table 19.1.

Functions of the spleen

The spleen is a specialized organ with an anatomical structure designed to allow antigens, which are circulating in the systemic bloodstream or have been absorbed from the gastrointestinal tract into the portal circulation, to be processed by macrophages of the RES and presented to the cells of the immune system. The functions of the spleen are therefore:

• processing of antigens to be presented to lymphoid cells;
• manufacture of antibody;
• phagocytosis of antibody-coated cells by the interaction with macrophages via their surface Fc receptors. The spleen is particularly important in protection against capsulated bacteria, e.g. *Pneumococcus* (see Chaper 19);
• to temporarily sequester red cells (especially reticulocytes) and remove nuclear remnants (Howell–Jolly bodies), siderotic (iron-containing) granules and other inclusions; and
• haemopoiesis in early fetal life; and (rarely) in some pathological states, e.g. chronic myelofibrosis.

Causes of splenomegaly are discussed in Chapter 19.

Haematology at a Glance, Fourth Edition. Atul B. Mehta and A. Victor Hoffbrand.

6.1 Immune thrombocytopenia: multiple bruises, ecchymoses and purpura

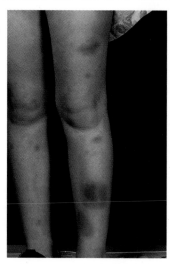

6.2 Thrombocytopenia: petechial rash

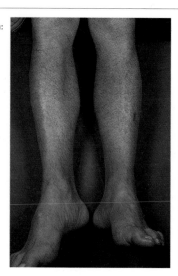

6.3 Physical signs in haematological disease

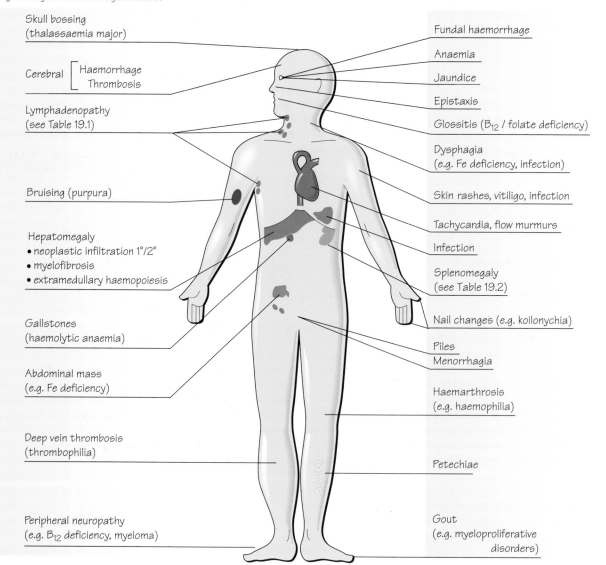

Skull bossing
(thalassaemia major)

Cerebral [Haemorrhage
Thrombosis

Lymphadenopathy
(see Table 19.1)

Bruising (purpura)

Hepatomegaly
• neoplastic infiltration 1°/2°
• myelofibrosis
• extramedullary haemopoiesis

Gallstones
(haemolytic anaemia)

Abdominal mass
(e.g. Fe deficiency)

Deep vein thrombosis
(thrombophilia)

Peripheral neuropathy
(e.g. B_{12} deficiency, myeloma)

Fundal haemorrhage

Anaemia

Jaundice

Epistaxis

Glossitis (B_{12} / folate deficiency)

Dysphagia
(e.g. Fe deficiency, infection)

Skin rashes, vitiligo, infection

Tachycardia, flow murmurs

Infection

Splenomegaly
(see Table 19.2)

Nail changes (e.g. koilonychia)

Piles
Menorrhagia

Haemarthrosis
(e.g. haemophilia)

Petechiae

Gout
(e.g. myeloproliferative
disorders)

Haematological illness leads to a range of symptoms and signs. An accurate history, careful clinical examination and appropriate laboratory assessment are essential for successful management of patients.

History

Anaemia
This is a reduction in the concentration of haemoglobin which leads to reduced oxygen carriage and delivery.
- Symptoms: shortness of breath on exertion, tiredness, headache or angina, more marked if anaemia is severe, of rapid onset and in older subjects.
- Causes: e.g. bleeding, dietary deficiency, malabsorption, systemic illness, haemolysis (i.e. accelerated destruction), bone marrow failure of red cell production.

Leucopenia
This is a reduction in white cell number which, if severe, predisposes to infection. It may be due to the following:
- Neutropenia, particularly if neutrophils are $<0.5 \times 10^9$/L, which frequently leads to bacterial or fungal infection in skin, mouth, throat and chest. Pus is lacking.
- Infection is often atypical, caused by organisms non-pathogenic for normal individuals, rapidly progressive and difficult to treat.
- Lymphopenia due to a reduction in B and/or T cell (humoral and T-cell-mediated) immunity predisposes particularly to viral infection (e.g. herpes zoster), tuberculosis, protozoal and fungal infections.
- Functional defects of neutrophils and lymphocytes also predispose to infection.

Thrombocytopenia
This is a reduction in blood platelets which, if severe, leads to spontaneous bruising and bleeding (Figs 6.1 and 6.2).
- Spontaneous bruises (purpura) may be raised (ecchymoses) or small pin-sized capillary haemorrhages (petechiae), mucosal bleeding, e.g. epistaxis, menorrhagia. Bleeding following trauma is increased with platelets $<50 \times 10^9$/L. Spontaneous bleeding occurs particularly when platelets $<10 \times 10^9$/L.
- Functional platelet defects also predispose to bleeding.
NB: Combination of anaemia, excessive bleeding and/or infection suggest pancytopenia caused by bone marrow failure (see Chapter 36).

Coagulation factor defects
- Easy bleeding after trauma (e.g. circumcision, dental treatment), spontaneous haemorrhage in deep tissues (e.g. muscles, joints).
- Family history is important in inherited defects, e.g. haemophilia.
- Acquired coagulation defects lead to spontaneous purpura and bleeding, with excessive bleeding in response to trauma.

Other symptoms
- Weight loss, fever, pruritus and skin rash – lymphoma or myeloproliferative disorder.
- Bone pain, symptoms of hypercalcaemia (thirst, polyuria, constipation) – myeloma.
- Left hypochondrial pain – splenomegaly.
- Painless lymphadenopathy suggests malignancy, whereas painful lymphadenopathy usually indicates inflammation/infection.
- Joint pains – gout caused by hyperuricaemia.

Family history
Inherited anaemia (e.g. genetic disorders of haemoglobin), coagulation disorders (e.g. haemophilia) and certain leucocyte and platelet disorders.

Drug history
Haemolytic anaemia in glucose 6-phosphate dehydrogenase (G6PD) deficiency (see Chapter 14), disordered platelet function caused by aspirin, drug-induced agranulocytosis, macrocytosis of red cells caused by alcohol.

Operations
Gastrectomy, intestinal resection may lead to iron or B_{12} deficiency. Splenectomy may lead to infection.

Examination (Fig. 6.3)
- Pallor of mucous membranes, if Hb <90 g/L, indicates anaemia.
- Tachycardia, systolic murmur (cardiac output and pulse rate rise to compensate for anaemia).
- Jaundice (haemolytic or megaloblastic anaemia), pigment gallstones.
- Lymphadenopathy (generalized or localized) (see Table 19.1).
- Skin changes, e.g. purpura caused by thrombocytopenia, vitiligo associated with pernicious anaemia, melanin pigmentation in iron overload, ankle ulcers in haemolytic anaemia, rashes caused by leukaemia or lymphoma infiltration.
- Nail changes (e.g. koilonychia in iron deficiency).
- Signs of infection (mouth, throat, skin, perineum, chest) associated with neutropenia. Fever may be the only sign.
- Mouth, e.g. angular cheilosis in iron deficiency, glossitis in B_{12} or folate deficiency.
- Hepatomegaly or splenomegaly (see Table 19.2).
- Nervous system examination, e.g. B_{12} neuropathy, peripheral neuropathy in myeloma, amyloidosis, malignant infiltration in central nervous system leukaemia or lymphoma.
- Optic fundi, e.g. haemorrhage in severe anaemia, hyperviscosity in polycythaemia.

Special investigations
Haematological diseases are often multisystem disorders and imaging investigations e.g. X-ray, ultrasound, CT/MRI are frequently required to define the extent and stage of the disease.

Nuclear medicine tests also useful to haematologists include the following:
- Positron emission tomography (PET) measures metabolic activity of tissue and is able to help stage lymphomas and to distinguish residual lymphoma (positive) from inactive scar tissue (negative) after chemotherapy or radiotherapy.
- Multiple gated acquisition (MUGA) scanning to assess left ventricular function (impaired due to chemotherapy, radiotherapy or iron overload).

Laboratory tests are described in Chapter 7.

7.1 Automated cell counter

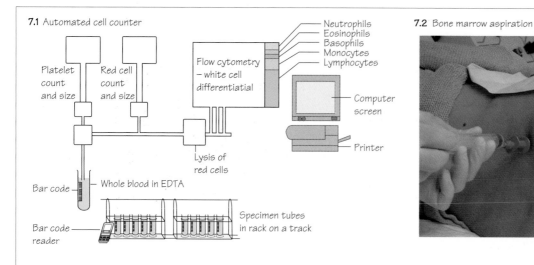

Platelet count and size

Red cell count and size

Flow cytometry – white cell differentiatial

Neutrophils
Eosinophils
Basophils
Monocytes
Lymphocytes

Computer screen

Printer

Lysis of red cells

Bar code — Whole blood in EDTA

Bar code reader

Specimen tubes in rack on a track

7.2 Bone marrow aspiration

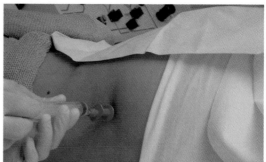

7.3 Low power microscopic view of bone marrow aspirate

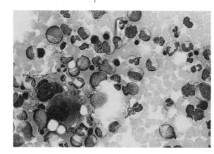

7.4 (i) Bone marrow trephine biopsy needle
(ii) Bone marrow aspirate needle

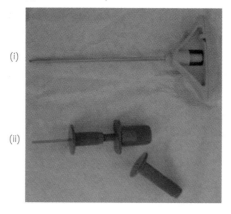

(i)

(ii)

7.5 Flow cytometry. In this example cells are simultaneously tested for CD34 and CD33 which are markers of myeloid differentiation. The patient suffers from acute myeloid leukaemia (AML)

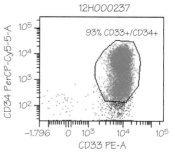

12H000237

93% CD33+/CD34+

AML M4 CD34+ CD33+

Haematology at a Glance, Fourth Edition. Atul B. Mehta and A. Victor Hoffbrand.

7.6 Chromosomal analysis : This example shows chromosomal analysis of the malignant cells from a patient with acute lymphoblastic leukaemia whose cells have a translocation of material (arrowed) from chromosome 4 to 11 (t4;11). This translocation is associated with a worse prognosis

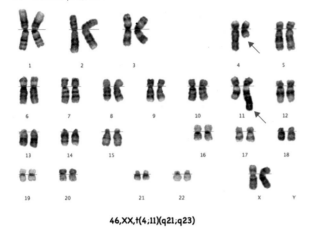

46,XX,t(4;11)(q21;q23)

7.7 Fluorescent *in situ* hybridization (FISH). Slides have been prepared from the cytogenetic preparation illustrated in 7.6. The probes for chromosomes 11 (red) and 4 (green) should be separate; however, it is clear that in a proportion of metaphases the signals sit alongside each other (t4;11)

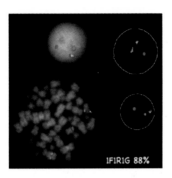

7.8 The polymerase chain reaction (PcR) to amplify DNA or RNA for further analysis

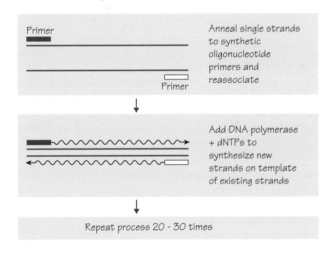

7.9 DNA microarray. DNA probes corresponding to different genes are immobilized in horizontal lanes. Fluorescent-labelled patient RNA or cDNA is added in vertical lanes. In this example, patients who subsequently responded to a new chemotherapy approach have a different pattern of gene expression to patients subsequently found to be non-responders

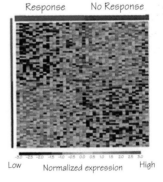

Routine tests

Full blood count (see Normal values Table 8.1)

Blood sample in sequestrene (ethylenediaminetetra-acetate, EDTA) anticoagulant is tested by an automated analyser. This counts the red cells and platelets after separation by size and the white cells after haemolysis of red cells (Fig. 7.1). The different white cells are counted according to their light refraction properties. Analysers provide the following:

• Haemoglobin concentration, haematocrit, red cell count, red cell indices (see Chapter 8)
• White cell count and differential (neutrophils, lymphocytes, monocytes; eosinophils and basophils)
• Platelet count and size

• Abnormal cells, e.g. nucleated red cells, myeloblasts, recorded as 'abnormal cells'
• Analysers also provide automated reticulocyte counts and enumerate immature platelets ('platelet reticulocytes').

Blood film

A *blood film* is made by spreading a drop of blood on a glass slide, staining with a Romanowsky stain, and examining the film microscopically, initially at low power and then at higher power (see Fig. 8.2). Most haematology laboratories make a blood film if specifically requested to do so by the clinician, for patients with a known haematological disorder and for new patients who have an abnormal full blood count (FBC).

Erythrocyte sedimentation rate, plasma/whole blood viscosity and C-reactive protein

The erythrocyte sedimentation rate (ESR) measures the rate of fall of a column of red cells in plasma in 1 hour. It is largely determined by plasma concentrations of proteins, especially fibrinogen and globulins. It is also raised in anaemia. Normal range rises with age. A raised ESR is a non-specific indicator of an acute phase response and is of value in monitoring inflammatory disease activity (e.g. rheumatoid arthritis). A raised ESR occurs in inflammatory disorders, infections, malignancy, myeloma, anaemia and pregnancy. The *plasma viscosity* gives comparable information but is less widely used. *Whole blood viscosity* is also influenced by the cell counts and is therefore raised when the red cell count (erythrocrit), white cell count (leucocrit) or platelet count is grossly raised. *C-reactive protein* is raised in an acute phase response, e.g. to infection, and is valuable in monitoring this.

Bone marrow aspiration

Bone marrow is aspirated from the posterior iliac crest; a trephine biopsy (see below) is usually taken at the same time. Alternative sites for aspiration of marrow are the sternum and the medial part of the tibia (infants). The procedure is performed under local anaesthesia with or without intravenous sedation (Fig. 7.2). Indications for marrow aspiration are listed in Box 7.1. Aspirated cells and particles of marrow are spread on slides (Fig. 7.3), stained by Romanowsky stain and for iron (Perls' stain; see Fig. 10.4). Specialized tests may also be performed (Box 7.2).

Bone marrow trephine biopsy

This is a more invasive procedure, using a larger needle (Fig. 7.4) whereby a core of bone is obtained from the iliac crest. This is then fixed in formalin and sections are cut. It is stained routinely by haematoxylin and eosin and a silver stain. Immunostaining is also performed if a haematological malignancy is suspected.

Specialized tests

Tests for the cause of anaemia are discussed in Chapter 8 and in the chapters dealing with different types of anaemia, e.g. iron deficiency, megaloblastic, haemolytic or haemoglobin disorders. The tests needed usually depend on the type of anaemia (microcytic, normocytic or macrocytic) and whether or not white cells and platelet abnormalities are also present. If so, bone marrow examination is most likely to be needed. The tests used particularly in diagnosis of malignant haematological diseases but also for some benign haematological disorders are described here.

Box 7.1 Indications for bone marrow aspiration (and trephine)*

- Unexplained cytopenia*
  Anaemia, leucopenia, thrombocytopenia
- Suspected marrow infiltrate*
  Leukaemia, myelodysplasia, lymphoma, myeloproliferative disease, myeloma, carcinoma, storage disorders
- Suspected infection
  Leishmaniasis, tuberculosis

*Bone marrow trephine is required for pancytopenia or suspected marrow infiltration

---

Box 7.2 Special tests on bone marrow cells: diagnosis and classification of haematological malignant diseases

Chromosomes
Conventional cytogenetics, e.g. diagnosis and classification of leukaemia, myelodysplasia

FISH
Sensitive detection of chromosome deletions, duplications, translocations, inversions

DNA analysis
Detection and classification of:
- leukaemia
- myeloproliferative diseases
- lymphoproliferative diseases
Detection of residual disease

Immunophenotype analysis
Diagnosis and classification of:
- leukaemia
- lymphoproliferative diseases
- detection of residual disease

Gene array analysis

Flow cytometry

Flow cytometry (Fig. 7.5) is an automated technique whereby a population of cells is incubated with specific monoclonal antibodies which are conjugated to a fluorochrome. The labelled cells are then passed in a fluid stream across a laser light source which allows quantitative analysis of antigen expression on the cell population. The technique is important in detecting and quantifying abnormal populations of cells, e.g. leukaemia diagnosis, assessment of residual malignant disease.

Chromosome analysis

Normal individuals have 46 chromosomes: 44 autosomes (22 from each parent) and 2 sex chromosomes (46 XY = male, 46 XX = female) in each somatic cell. Chromosomal analysis is made initially by special stains of cells in division. Loss or gain of whole chromosomes, chromosome breaks and loss, inversion or translocation of a part of a chromosome can be detected (Fig. 7.6).

Fluorescent *in situ* hybridization (FISH) is a more sensitive technique for detecting chromosome abnormalities (Fig. 7.7). It involves the use of a fluorescent DNA probe that hybridizes selectively to a particular chromosome segment, allowing sensitive microscopic detection of deletion, translocation and duplication of that segment, or fusion with another chromosome. It has the advantage not only of detecting small abnormalities, but being applicable to interphase (non-dividing) cells.

DNA (genetic) abnormalities

A DNA or genetic abnormality as a cause of haematological disease may be inherited or acquired. *Inherited* haematological diseases are most commonly autosomal recessive, requiring an individual to inherit two mutant copies (alleles) of a gene (one from each parent) for expression of the disease (homozygotes). Carriers (heterozygotes) have one normal and one mutant allele and may express no or minor abnormalities clinically, e.g. sickle cell trait. Autosomal dominant diseases, e.g. hereditary spherocytosis, are rarer and require only one mutant allele for full expression of the disease. Sex-linked diseases, e.g. haemophilia, arise if the mutant gene is on the X chromosome; males, having only one X chromosome (hemizygous), are affected, whereas females are carriers. *Acquired* DNA abnormalities are frequently present in clones of malignant cell populations and serve as disease markers and clues to pathogenesis (see Chapter 20).

Molecular techniques

• Polymerase chain reaction (PCR) (Fig. 7.8) can be used to amplify a DNA segment which can then be sequenced or digested by a restriction enzyme and fractionated by size using gel electrophoresis. PCR can be used to detect a DNA point mutation, e.g. of JAK2 (see Chapter 26) which may underlie a haematological disease. It can also be used to characterize a clone of malignant cells (minimal residual disease;

see Chapter 20). PCR is also used to diagnose inherited mutations (e.g. of haemoglobin and of coagulation proteins) and it is used widely for antenatal diagnosis. PCR can be quantitative, e.g. 'real time', in which the number of cycles required to give a certain amount of DNA is compared with a known standard.

New ('second generation') sequencing techniques allowing rapid whole genome sequencing are revealing new clonal point mutations underlying various haematological malignancies e.g. AML, MDS, CLL.

• Gene expression is studied by analysing RNA extracted from fresh cells, e.g. by gel electrophoresis (Northern blot). It can be semi-quantitated by using the enzyme reverse transcriptase to generate a DNA copy and then applying a modified PCR technique.

• DNA microarrays analyse expression of multiple cellular genes (Fig. 7.9). Fluorescent-labelled cell RNA or cDNA to be analysed is hybridized to DNA probes immobilized on a solid support. The pattern of mRNA expression is obtained, and this is characteristic of the leukaemia or lymphoma subtype or prognostic group. Microarrays can also be used to detect small deletions or gains in DNA.

8.1 Printout of a normal blood count from a 34-year-old Caucasian female

Test	Results	Range
Hb	133 g/L	115–155
WBC	7.43 10^9/L	3.5–11
Platelets	236 10^9/L	140–400
RBC	4.68 10^{12}/L	3.9–5.4
HCT	0.407 L/L	0.35–0.47
MCV	87.0 fL	80–98
MCH	28.4 pg	27–33
MCHC	32.7 g/dL	31–37
Neutrophils	4.09 10^9/L	1.7–8.0
Lymphocytes	2.54 10^9/L	1.0–3.5
Monocytes	0.64 10^9/L	0.1–1.0
Eosinophils	0.13 10^9/L	0.0–0.46
Basophils	0.03 10^9/L	0.00–0.20

8.2 Normal blood film (low power, × 25 magnification) showing normal red cells. Platelets (arrow A), a normal neutrophil (arrow B), and a lymphocyte (arrow C). A normal monocyte (arrow D), eosinophil (arrow E) and basophil (arrow F) are also illustrated

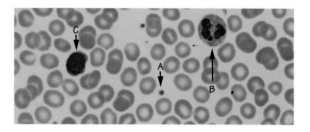

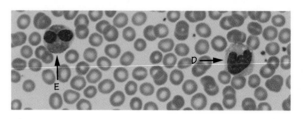

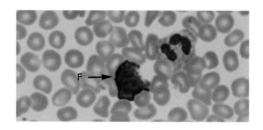

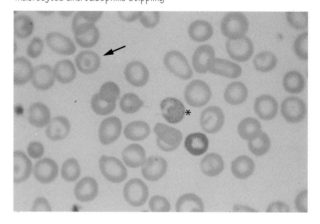

8.3 Leucoerythroblastic blood film showing circulating immature granulocytes and a nucleated red blood cell indicating in this case marrow infiltration by carcinoma

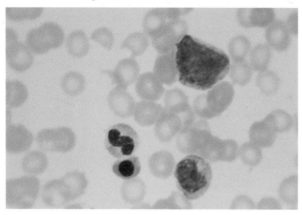

8.4 Renal failure: peripheral blood film showing irregular red cells ('burr cells') (arrows), fragmented red cells and a neutrophil showing toxic granulation and vacuolation

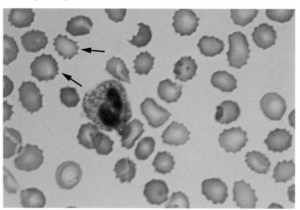

8.5 Liver disease: peripheral blood film showing target cells (arrow), macrocytes and basophilic stippling*

Haematology at a Glance, Fourth Edition. Atul B. Mehta and A. Victor Hoffbrand.

Anaemia

Anaemia is defined as a reduction in haemoglobin concentration below the normal range for the age and sex of the individual. It is usually accompanied by a reduction in red cell count and haematocrit.

Clinical features

Symptoms of anaemia are mainly shortness of breath on exertion, tiredness and headaches. If it is severe in older people, congestive heart failure or angina may develop. There is a rise in red cell 2,3-diphosphoglycerate (2,3-DPG) in most cases of anaemia so that oxygen is given up more readily to tissues. The main signs are pallor of the mucous membranes if the haemoglobin is <90 g/L with increased cardiac output shown by tachycardia and possibly a systolic murmur. Signs associated with particular forms of anaemia, e.g. jaundice in haemolytic or megaloblastic anaemia, koilonychia in iron deficiency, may be present and these are described with the individual anaemias.

Investigations

Anaemia is not, by itself, a sufficient diagnosis. Further assessment must be undertaken to establish the cause before treatment can be given (Box 8.1). This is done by clinical assessment (history, physical examination) and appropriate use of special investigations. A classification of anaemia according to whether red cells are large (macrocytic) or small (microcytic) is used to guide further investigations (Box 8.2) and further details on the specific types of anaemia are given in the appropriate chapters.

The *full blood count (FBC)* must be performed as an initial investigation using an automatic cell counter. The red cell indices (mean corpuscular volume, MCV; mean corpuscular haemoglobin, MCH) and red cell count (RBC $\times$ 10^{12}/L) give indicators of the type of anaemia (e.g. microcytic or macrocytic). A printout of a normal blood count from an automated analyser is illustrated (Fig. 8.1a). The blood count and film will also reveal any white cell or platelet abnormalities. If all three types of blood cell are abnormal, a bone marrow defect is likely. Pancytopenia is used to describe subclinical levels of haemoglobin, neutrophils and platelets.

A *stained blood film* is made for examining red cell morphology as a clue to underlying pathology (Fig. 8.2). The blood film also allows estimation of the white cell differential count, although this is now usually performed automatically by the cell counter. The blood film also allows examination of morphology of white cells, platelets, for presence of abnormal cells (e.g. normoblasts) and for any circulating non-haemopoietic cells (e.g. malarial parasites).

Haemoglobin disorders (see Chapters 16 and 17) are among the most common inherited conditions. Haemoglobin electrophoresis is a simple technique to separate different haemoglobins. Red cells are lysed to release haemoglobin, and the lysate is applied to a gel across which an electric current is applied (see Fig. 16.6). High performance liquid chromatography (HPLC) is an increasingly used automated technique used in place of haemoglobin electrophoresis (see Fig 16.5). These techniques are used to detect an abnormal haemoglobin, and to determine the relative proportions of the different normal haemoglobins (Hb A, A_2, F).

Haematinic levels (i.e. serum B_{12}, folate, ferritin, iron and iron-binding capacity) are performed by analysers using immunoassay. The results may indicate the underlying cause of anaemia.

Some common anaemias that occur with systemic diseases are described next.

Box 8.1 Causes of anaemia

Inherited

Usually associated with reduced red cell survival (haemolytic anaemias):

- Defects of haemoglobin, e.g. sickle cell, thalassaemia
- Defects of red cell metabolism, e.g. pyruvate kinase deficiency
- Defects of red cell membrane, e.g. hereditary spherocytosis
- Red cell aplasia/aplastic anaemia

Acquired

Reduced red cell production due to:

- Haematinic deficiency (iron, B_{12}, folate, B_6)
- Marrow replacement, e.g. by tumour (leukaemia, myeloma, lymphoma)
- Marrow aplasia

Increased red cell destruction (haemolytic anaemia) due to:

- Immune destruction
- Red cell fragmentation syndromes
- Chemical and physical agents
- Infections
- Paroxysmal nocturnal haemoglobinuria

Systemic illnesses:

- Anaemia of chronic disease
- Renal failure, liver, cardiac, endocrine disease

Box 8.2 Classification of anaemia according to red cell size

Macrocytic (MCV >98 fl)

Megaloblastic
  B_{12} or folate deficiency
Other
  See Box 12.1

Normocytic (MCV = 78–98 fl)

Most haemolytic anaemias
Anaemia of chronic disorders (some cases)
Mixed cases

Microcytic (MCV <78 fl; MCH usually also <27 pg/L)

Iron deficiency
Thalassaemia (α or β)
Other haemoglobin defects
Anaemia of chronic disorders (some cases)
Congenital sideroblastic anaemia (rare)

MCH, mean cell haemoglobin; MCV, mean cell volume

Anaemia of chronic disease

- Anaemia of chronic disease (ACD) is a common normochromic or mildly hypochromic anaemia, occurring in patients with different inflammatory and malignant diseases (Box 8.3).
- Moderate anaemia occurs, haemoglobin level >90 g/L, severity of anaemia correlating with severity of underlying disease.
- Reduced serum iron and total iron-binding capacity.

Chronic infections

Especially osteomyelitis, bacterial endocarditis, tuberculosis, chronic abscesses, bronchiectasis, chronic urinary tract infections, HIV, AIDS, malaria

Other chronic inflammatory disorders

Rheumatoid arthritis, polymyalgia rheumatica, systemic lupus erythematosus, scleroderma, inflammatory bowel disease, thrombophlebitis

Malignant diseases

Carcinoma, especially metastatic or associated with infection, lymphoma

Others

Congestive heart failure

• Normal or raised serum ferritin with adequate iron stores in the bone marrow but stainable iron absent from erythroblasts.
• Usually, the erythrocyte sedimentation rate and C-reactive protein are raised.

Pathogenesis

Hepcidin, released by the liver in response to inflammatory cytokines, e.g. interleukin 6 (IL-6), reduces iron absorption and iron release by macrophages into plasma. Increased levels of cytokines, especially IL-1, IL-6, tumour necrosis factor and interferon-γ, also interact directly with accessory marrow stromal cells, macrophages and erythroid progenitors to reduce erythropoiesis, iron utilization and response to erythropoietin (EPO).

Treatment

• Therapy of the chronic disease gradually reduces levels of mediator cytokines.
• Recombinant EPO may improve anaemia in patients with, e.g. rheumatoid arthritis (RA), cancer and myeloma.

Malignancy
Anaemia

• ACD affects almost all cancer patients at some stage.
• Blood loss in gastrointestinal and gynaecological malignancies.
• Autoimmune haemolytic anaemia, especially in lymphoma.
• Microangiopathic haemolytic anaemia (see Chapter 15) may occur with disseminated mucin-secreting adenocarcinoma.
• Leucoerythroblastic anaemia indicates marrow infiltration by tumour (Fig. 8.3).

• Red cell aplasia is associated with thymoma, lymphoma and chronic lymphocytic leukaemia.
• Chemotherapy or radiotherapy-induced inhibition of bone marrow.
• Folate deficiency as a result of poor diet and widespread disease.

Connective tissue disorders
Anaemia

• ACD is common. Iron deficiency may coexist in patients with gastrointestinal haemorrhage caused by non-steroidal anti-inflammatory agents.
• Autoimmune haemolytic anaemia occurs in systemic lupus erythematosus (SLE), RA and mixed connective tissue disorders.
• Red cell aplasia occurs in SLE.

Renal disease
Anaemia

Acute or chronic renal failure causes a normochromic normocytic anaemia, with reduced EPO levels – the main cause of anaemia – and echinocytes (burr cells) in the blood film (Fig. 8.4). Iron deficiency (blood loss) and haemolysis in the haemolytic uraemic syndrome and thrombotic thrombocytopenic purpura are other causes. EPO corrects anaemia up to a haemoglobin level of 120 g/L. A poor response to EPO occurs with iron or folate deficiency, haemolysis, infection, occult malignancy, aluminium toxicity, hyperparathyroidism and inadequate dialysis. Hypertension and thrombosis of an arteriovenous fistula may occur with EPO therapy.

Polycythaemia

Polycythaemia may occur with renal tumours or cysts, leading to excess production of EPO.

Endocrine disease
Anaemia

Both hyper- and hypothyroidism cause mild anaemia (MCV raised in hypothyroidism, low in thyrotoxicosis). Deficiencies of iron, as a result of menorrhagia or achlorhydria, or of B_{12} (increased incidence of pernicious anaemia in hypothyroidism, hypoadrenalism and hypoparathyroidism), may complicate the anaemia. Antithyroid drugs (carbimazole and propylthiouracil) can cause aplastic anaemia or agranulocytosis.

Liver disease
Anaemia

This may be caused by anaemia of chronic disease, haemodilution (increased plasma volume), pooling of red cells (splenomegaly) and haemorrhage, e.g. caused by oesophageal varices. The MCV is raised, particularly in alcoholics, and target cells, echinocytes and acanthocytes occur in the blood film (Fig. 8.5). Haemolysis and hypertriglyceridaemia with alcoholic liver disease (Zieve syndrome) is rare. Direct toxicity of copper for red cells causes haemolysis in Wilson disease. Viral hepatitis, including hepatitis A, B and C and hepatitis viruses yet to be characterized, may lead to aplastic anaemia.

9 Iron I: physiology and deficiency

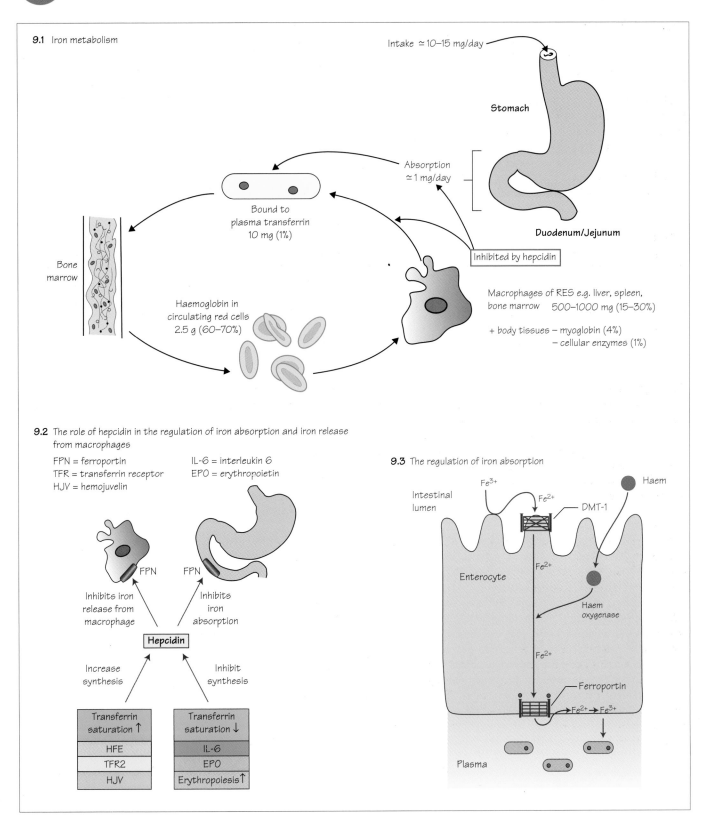

9.1 Iron metabolism

Intake ≃ 10–15 mg/day

Stomach

Duodenum/Jejunum

Absorption ≃ 1 mg/day

Inhibited by hepcidin

Bound to plasma transferrin 10 mg (1%)

Bone marrow

Haemoglobin in circulating red cells 2.5 g (60–70%)

Macrophages of RES e.g. liver, spleen, bone marrow 500–1000 mg (15–30%)

+ body tissues – myoglobin (4%)
– cellular enzymes (1%)

9.2 The role of hepcidin in the regulation of iron absorption and iron release from macrophages

FPN = ferroportin
TFR = transferrin receptor
HJV = hemojuvelin
IL-6 = interleukin 6
EPO = erythropoietin

FPN

FPN

Inhibits iron release from macrophage

Inhibits iron absorption

Hepcidin

Increase synthesis

Inhibit synthesis

Transferrin saturation ↑	Transferrin saturation ↓
HFE	IL-6
TFR2	EPO
HJV	Erythropoiesis ↑

9.3 The regulation of iron absorption

Intestinal lumen

Fe^{3+}

Fe^{2+}

DMT-1

Haem

Enterocyte

Fe^{2+}

Haem oxygenase

Fe^{2+}

Ferroportin

$Fe^{2+} \rightarrow Fe^{3+}$

Plasma

Haematology at a Glance, Fourth Edition. Atul B. Mehta and A. Victor Hoffbrand.

9.4 Nail changes in chronic iron deficiency include brittle nails, ridged nails and spoon-shaped nails (koilonychia)

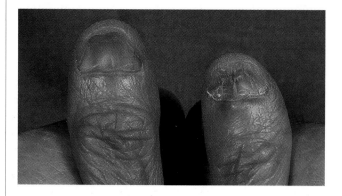

9.5 Iron deficiency. Peripheral blood film showing hypochromic microcytic cells, with variation in cell size (anisocytosis) and abnormally shaped cells (poikilocytosis)

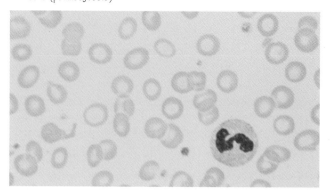

9.6 Serum iron, unsaturated serum iron-binding capacity (UIBC) and serum ferritin in normal subjects and in those with iron deficiency, anaemia of chronic disorders and iron overload

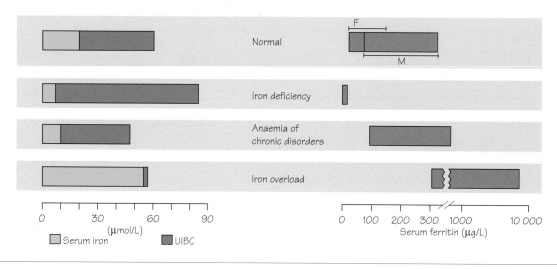

Distribution of body iron

Iron is contained in haemoglobin, the reticuloendothelial system (as ferritin and haemosiderin), muscle (myoglobin), plasma (bound to transferrin) and cellular enzymes (e.g. cytochromes, catalase) (Fig. 9.1). Reticuloendothelial cells (macrophages) gain iron from the haemoglobin of effete red cells and release it to plasma transferrin which transports iron to bone marrow and other tissues with transferrin receptors (TFRs).

Hepcidin

Hepcidin is a protein synthesized by the liver that controls iron absorption and circulation (Fig. 9.2). It lowers cell levels of ferroportin, the protein that allows iron entry into the portal circulation (Fig. 9.3) from the duodenal enterocytes and into the blood circulation from macrophages. Hepcidin therefore reduces both iron absorption and iron release from macrophages to transferrin. Hepcidin synthesis is controlled by various proteins, e.g. HFE, hemojuvelin (HJV) and the minor transferrin receptor TFR2. Mutation of any of these lowers hepcidin secretion and causes excess iron absorption (see Chapter 10). Inflam-

mation increases hepcidin synthesis through increased levels of IL-6. Increased iron stores stimulate hepcidin synthesis while iron deficiency reduces it. Increased erythropoiesis lowers hepcidin synthesis because of a protein GDF15 released from erythroblasts.

Iron intake, absorption and loss

The average Western diet contains 10–15 mg/day of iron, of which 5–10% (about 1 mg) is normally absorbed through the upper small intestine. Absorption is normally adjusted to body needs (increased in iron deficiency and pregnancy, reduced in iron overload). Absorption is regulated by DMT-1 at the villous tip and ferroportin (controlled by hepcidin) at the basolateral surface of the enterocyte (Fig. 9.3). At the luminal surface iron is reduced to the Fe^{2+} state and on entry to portal plasma reoxidized to Fe^{3+}. It then binds to transferrin. Haem from food is degraded after absorption through the cell surface to release Fe^{2+}. Some iron remains in the enterocyte as ferritin.

Iron in animal products is more easily absorbed than vegetable iron; inorganic iron in ferrous form is absorbed more easily than ferric form. Vitamin C enhances absorption; phytates inhibit it. Dietary intake makes up for daily loss (about 1 mg) in hair, skin, urine, faeces and menstrual blood loss in women. Infants, children and pregnant women need extra iron to expand their red cell mass and, in pregnancy, for transfer to the fetus.

Iron deficiency

Causes (Box 9.1)

• Blood loss (500 mL of normal blood contains 200–250 mg iron) – the dominant cause in Western countries.
• Malabsorption – rarely a main cause.
• Poor dietary intake – may be a contributory cause, especially in children, menstruating females or pregnancy; a major factor in developing countries.

Clinical features

• General features of anaemia (see Chapter 8).
• Special features (minority of patients): koilonychia (Fig. 9.4) or ridged brittle nails, glossitis, angular cheilosis (sore corners of mouth),

---

pica (abnormal appetite), hair thinning and pharyngeal web formation (Paterson–Kelly syndrome).
• Features resulting from an underlying cause of haemorrhage.
  NB: Iron deficiency is the most common cause of anaemia in all countries of the world.

Laboratory findings

• Hypochromic microcytic anaemia.
• Raised platelet count.
• Blood film appearances (Fig. 9.5) include hypochromic/microcytic cells, anisocytosis/poikilocytosis, target cells and 'pencil' cells.
• Bone marrow – not needed for diagnosis: erythroblasts show ragged irregular cytoplasm; absence of iron from stores and erythroblasts (detected by Perls' stain).
• Serum ferritin reduced, serum iron low with raised transferrin and reduced saturation of iron-binding capacity (Fig. 9.6).

Other investigations

• History (especially for blood loss, diet, malabsorption). Tests for cause (especially in males and postmenopausal females) include occult blood tests, upper and lower gastrointestinal endoscopy, capsule (camera) endoscopy, tests for hookworm, malabsorption and urine haemosiderin.
• Haemoglobin high performance liquid chromatography (HPLC) or electrophoresis (see Chapter 16) and/or globin gene DNA analysis to exclude thalassaemia trait or other haemoglobin defect causing a microcytic hypochromic blood picture.

Treatment

• Oral iron – ferrous sulfate is best (200 mg, 67 mg iron per tablet) before meals three times daily.
• A reticulocyte response begins in 7 days, but treatment should be continued for 4–6 months to replenish stores.
• Side effects (e.g. abdominal pain, diarrhoea or constipation) require a lower dose, taking iron with food, or a different preparation (e.g. ferrous gluconate 300 mg, 37 mg iron per tablet).
• Poor response may be because of continued bleeding, incorrect diagnosis, malabsorption or poor compliance.
• Oral iron, often combined with folic acid, is given for iron deficiency in pregnancy.
• Intravenous iron is used in patients with malabsorption or who are unable to take oral iron. Ferric hydroxyide sucrose (Venofer), iron dextran (Cosmofer), ferric carboxymaltose (Ferinject) and iron isomaltoside (Monofer) are useful to treat iron deficiency anaemia and replenish iron stores. In the United States ferumoxytol (Feraheme) is also used.

> ## Box 9.1 Causes of iron deficiency
>
> ### Chronic blood loss
> Uterine, e.g. menorrhagia or postmenopausal bleeding
> Gastrointestinal, e.g. oesophageal varices, hiatus hernia, atrophic gastritis, *Helicobacter* infection, peptic ulcer, ingestion of aspirin (or other non-steroidal anti-inflammatory drugs), gastrectomy, carcinoma (stomach, caecum, colon or rectum), hookworm, angiodysplasia, colitis, diverticulosis, piles
> Rarely, haematuria, haemoglobinuria, pulmonary haemosiderosis, self-inflicted blood loss
>
> ### Increased demands
> Prematurity
> Growth*
> Pregnancy*
>
> ### Malabsorption
> Postgastrectomy, gluten-induced enteropathy, autoimmune gastritis
>
> ### Poor diet
> Rarely the sole cause in developed countries
>
> *Deficiency occurs if these are associated with poor diet

10.1 Iron overload: clinical features

Endocrine changes

Hypopituitarism

Hypothyroidism

Hypoparathyroidism

Excessive melanin
skin pigmentation
('bronze diabetes')

Cardiomyopathy

Cirrhosis/haemosiderosis
of liver

Diabetes mellitus

Ovarian or testicular
failure

Arthropathy in genetic
haemochromatosis

Delayed puberty
and secondary
sexual characteristics

10.2 Cardiovascular magnetic resonance T2* images showing the heart and liver from 3 different patients at the same echo time : A. Normal appearance with a bright myocardial and liver signal indicating that there is no significant cardiac or hepatic iron loading. B. Dark myocardial signal indicating severe myocardial siderosis but no liver iron. Note that the spleen (asterisk) also has high signal, suggesting that there is no significant splenic iron loading. C. Normal myocardial signal but dark liver consistent with severe hepatic iron overload. Images courtesy of Dr J.P. Carpenter from Hoffbrand AV et al. Blood 2012; 120. Reproduced with permission of John Wiley & Sons, Ltd

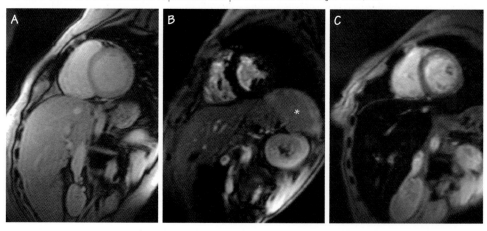

10.3 Bone marrow iron stain (Perls' stain, Prussian blue) showing a ringed sideroblast

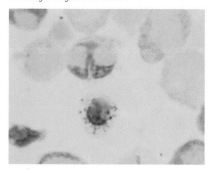

10.4 Basophilic stippling in red cells of a patient with lead poisoning

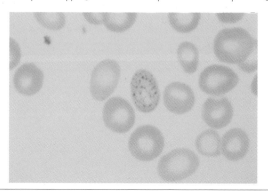

Iron overload

Iron overload is the pathological state in which total body stores of iron are increased, often with organ dysfunction as a result of iron deposition.

Causes

• Primary (genetic) haemochromatosis (GH) is an autosomal recessive condition associated with excessive iron absorption. Ninety per cent of cases are homozygous for a mutation in the *HFE* gene. Rarely, GH is caused by mutation of the hepcidin, hemojuvelin, or transferrin receptor 2 gene. All these proteins are involved in hepcidin synthesis (see Fig. 9.2) and all cases show low serum levels of hepcidin.
• African iron overload; dietary and genetic components.
• Excess dietary iron.
• Ineffective erythropoiesis with increased iron absorption (e.g. thalassaemia intermedia) due to inappropriately low levels of hepcidin.
• Repeated blood transfusions in patients with severe refractory anaemia, e.g. thalassaemia major, myelodysplasia. Each unit of blood contains 200–250 mg iron.

Clinical features

• These are mainly caused by organ dysfunction as a result of iron deposition (Fig. 10.1).
• Cardiomyopathy gives rise to dysrhythmias and congestive heart failure, major causes of death.
• Growth/sexual development is reduced in children; delayed puberty, diabetes mellitus, hypothyroidism and hypoparathyroidism are frequent.
• The liver may show haemosiderosis or cirrhosis. The liver abnormality in transfusional iron overload is, however, often a result of hepatitis B or C infection. Hepatocellular carcinoma is a complication of cirrhosis.
• Excessive melanin skin pigmentation.
• Excessive infections.
• Arthropathy in genetic haemochromatosis caused by pyrophosphate deposition.

Laboratory features

• Raised serum iron and transferrin saturation.
• Raised serum ferritin.
• Increased iron in liver (histology, chemical or MRI estimation).
• Abnormal liver function tests. Alpha-fetoprotein, an indicator of hepatocellular carcinoma, is tested regularly if cirrhosis is present.
• Increased urinary iron excretion in response to iron chelator therapy.
• Cardiomyopathy causes abnormal echocardiographic findings, e.g. reduced left ventricular ejection fraction or arrhythmia.
• MRI is used to measure tissue iron. The T_2* technique is best to measure liver and heart iron simultaneously (Fig. 10.2). It may detect iron excess in the heart before clinical or echocardiographic abnormalities.
• Endocrine abnormalities, e.g. raised blood glucose, low testosterone, oestrogen or pituitary hormone levels.

Treatment

• Genetic haemochromatosis: regular venesections to reduce iron level to normal, assessed by serum ferritin, serum iron and total iron-binding capacity and by liver biopsy or MRI.
• Transfusional iron overload: iron chelation is described in Chapter 16.

Sideroblastic anaemia

Definition

Sideroblastic anaemia is a refractory anaemia in which the marrow shows iron present as granules arranged in a ring around the nucleus in developing erythroblasts ('ringed sideroblasts'; Fig. 10.4). At least 15% of erythroblasts show this in the primary forms. A defect of haem synthesis is present.

Classification

• The most common form is the primary acquired type (a type of myelodysplasia; see Chapter 25).
• An X-linked genetic defect in haem synthesis, usually caused by mutation of δ-amino laevulinic acid synthase (ALA-S), a key enzyme in haem synthesis, underlies most congenital forms. These occur predominantly in males.
• Ringed sideroblasts (less than 15%) may also occur with other haematological disorders and with alcohol, isoniazid therapy and lead poisoning.

Clinical and laboratory features

The congenital anaemia is sometimes mild (haemoglobin 80–100 g/L) but may become more severe with age. The blood film is often hypochromic microcytic. Leucopenia and thrombocytopenia may occur in patients with myelodysplasia. The mean corpuscular volume is usually low in the inherited variety but raised in myelodysplasia.

Treatment

Usually symptomatic. Regular blood transfusion and iron chelation are often required. Patients with inherited forms may respond to pyridoxine (vitamin B_6), a cofactor for ALA-S.

Lead poisoning

Clinically, this presents with abdominal pain, constipation, anaemia, peripheral neuropathy and a blue (lead) line of the gums. The blood film shows punctate basophilia (blue staining dots as a result of undegraded RNA) (Fig. 10.5) and features of haemolysis. The marrow may show ringed sideroblasts.

Acute iron poisoning

This is most common in childhood and is usually accidental. Clinical features include nausea, abdominal pain, diarrhoea, gastrointestinal bleeding and abnormalities of liver function. Immediate treatment is with gastric lavage (within 1–2 hours); whole bowel irrigation may be indicated. Intravenous desferrioxamine is valuable in chelating iron and reducing risk of liver damage.

Megaloblastic anaemia I: vitamin B₁₂ (B₁₂) and folate deficiency – biochemical basis, causes

11.1 The role of vitamin B₁₂ in conversion of 5-methyltetrahydrofolate (methyl-THF) to tetrahydrofolate (THF) required as substrate for folate polyglutamate coenzyme synthesis, needed for DNA synthesis

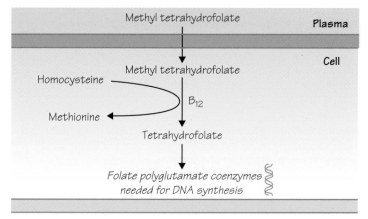

11.2 The gastrointestinal tract in B₁₂ or folate deficiency

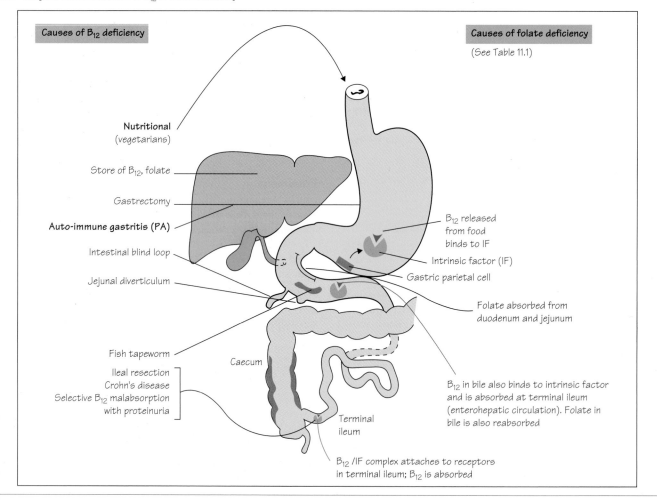

Haematology at a Glance, Fourth Edition. Atul B. Mehta and A. Victor Hoffbrand.

Megaloblastic anaemia is characterised by an abnormal appearance of the bone marrow erythroblasts in which nuclear development is delayed and nuclear chromatin has a lacy open appearance (Fig. 12.3). There is a defect in DNA synthesis usually caused by deficiency of vitamin B_{12} (B_{12}, cobalamin) or folate.

Biochemical basis

Folate is an essential coenzyme for the synthesis of thymidine monophosphate (TMP) and therefore of DNA because thymine is one of the four bases needed to form DNA. B_{12} is a coenzyme for methionine synthase, a reaction needed for the activation of folate. Demethylation of 5-methyl-tetrahydrofolate (methyl-THF) provides THF which acts as substrate for synthesis of intracellular folate polyglutamates which are coenzymes needed for DNA synthesis. During DNA synthesis (Fig. 11.1), folates are oxidized to the dihydrofolate form, and the enzyme dihydrofolate reductase (inhibited by methotrexate) is required to restore them to the active THF state.

B_{12} physiology (Fig. 11.2)

• Adult daily requirement for B_{12} is 1 µg (normal mixed diet contains 10–15 µg). B_{12} is present only in foods of animal origin: meat, fish, eggs, milk and butter; it is absent from vegetables, cereals and fruit, unless these are contaminated by microorganisms. Normal body stores of B_{12} are largely in the liver with an enterohepatic circulation. Stores are sufficient to last for 2–4 years.
• Dietary B_{12} combines with intrinsic factor (IF) secreted by gastric parietal cells (GPC). IF–B_{12} complex attaches to ileal receptors and B_{12} is absorbed.
• Absorbed B_{12} attaches to transcobalamin (TC) II which carries B_{12} in plasma to the liver, bone marrow, brain and other tissues. Most B_{12} in plasma is, however, attached to a second B_{12}-binding protein, TC I, and is functionally inactive.
• Passive absorption (about 0.1% of oral B_{12}) occurs through buccal, gastric and duodenal mucosae.

Causes of B_{12} deficiency (Fig. 11.2)

Inadequate diet

Vegans may develop B_{12} deficiency, although the intact enterohepatic circulation of a few micrograms of B_{12} daily delays its onset. Infants born to B_{12}-deficient mothers and breastfed by them may present with failure to thrive and megaloblastic anaemia resulting from B_{12} deficiency.

Malabsorption

Gastric causes

• Pernicious anaemia (PA) is the dominant cause of B_{12} deficiency in Western countries. It is characterized by an autoimmune gastritis, and reduced gastric secretion of IF and acid, and raised serum gastrin. It is often associated with other organ-specific autoimmune diseases (e.g. myxoedema, thyrotoxicosis, vitiligo, Addison disease and hypoparathyroidism). Antibodies to IF and gastric parietal cells occur in serum (50% and 90%, respectively) of patients. PA is also associated with early greying of hair, blue eyes, blood group A, a family history of PA or related autoimmune disease and a two- to threefold increased incidence of carcinoma of the stomach. It occurs in all races and has a female:male incidence of 1.6:1. Peak age of incidence is 60 years.
• Gastrectomy (total or subtotal) leads to B_{12} deficiency.
• Congenital IF deficiency or abnormality is rare.

Intestinal causes

These include bacterial (rarely fish tapeworm) colonization of small intestine, stagnant loop syndromes, congenital and acquired defects of the ileum (e.g. ileal resection, Crohn disease). Congenital B_{12} malabsorption with proteinuria (due to a genetic defect of the ileal receptor) is rare.

Less severe malabsorption of food B_{12} may occur with atrophic gastritis, *Helicobacter* infection, gluten-induced enteropathy and drugs, e.g. metformin.

Folate physiology

Folates consist of a large number of compounds derived from the parent compound pteroylglutamic (folic) acid by reduction, addition of single carbon groups, e.g. methyl or formyl, and, in cells, addition of extra glutamate moieties usually four, five or six to form polyglutamates.
• Folates occur in most foods, especially liver and green vegetables. Normal daily diet contains 200–250 µg, of which about 50% is absorbed.
• Daily adult requirements are about 100 µg; body stores are sufficient for 4 months.
• Absorbed through the upper small intestine with conversion of all natural forms to methyl-THF. A specific protein is needed for absorption of all forms of folate. An enterohepatic circulation exists.

Causes of folate deficiency (Box 11.1)

• The most common cause is poor dietary intake, either alone or in association with increased folate utilization (e.g. pregnancy or haemolytic anaemia).
• Malabsorption occurs in gluten-induced enteropathy or tropical sprue.
• Increased utilization: increased cell turnover and DNA synthesis causes breakdown of folates. The most common causes include pregnancy, haemolytic anaemia, severe chronic inflammatory and malignant diseases.
• Folate is loosely bound to protein in plasma and is easily removed by dialysis.

Box 11.1 Causes of folate deficiency

Nutritional
Especially old age, institutions, poverty, famine

Malabsorption
Gluten-induced enteropathy, dermatitis herpetiformis, tropical sprue

Excess utilization
Physiological:
• Pregnancy and lactation, prematurity
  Pathological:
• Haematological diseases: haemolytic anaemias, myelofibrosis
• Malignant diseases: carcinoma, lymphoma, myeloma
• Inflammatory diseases: Crohn disease, rheumatoid arthritis, extensive psoriasis, exfoliative dermatitis, malaria

Excess urinary folate loss
Congestive heart failure, chronic dialysis

Drugs
Anticonvulsants, sulfasalazine

Mixed
Liver disease, alcoholism (spirit drinkers)

---

12 Megaloblastic anaemia II: clinical features, treatment and other macrocytic anaemias

12.1 Pernicious anaemia in an elderly male. There is a tinge of jaundice and his skin is pale

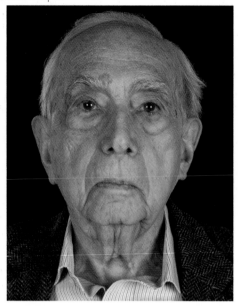

12.2 Peripheral blood in megaloblastic anaemia, showing a hypersegmented neutrophil (A), oval macrocytes and poikilocytosis (variation in red cell shape)

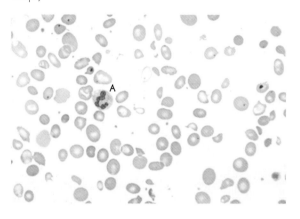

12.3 (a) Bone marrow in megaloblastic anaemia showing megaloblasts. These are nucleated erythroid cells with open lacy chromatin and delayed nuclear maturation. (b) Megaloblasts with developing myeloid cells; the cell with a C-shaped nucleus (arrow) is a giant metamyelocyte

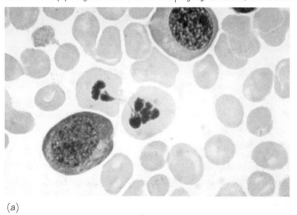

(a)

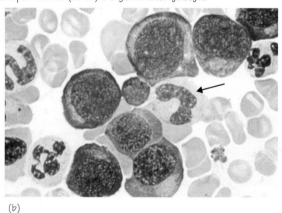

(b)

Haematology at a Glance, Fourth Edition. Atul B. Mehta and A. Victor Hoffbrand.

40 © 2014 John Wiley & Sons, Ltd. Published 2014 by John Wiley & Sons, Ltd. Companion Website: www.ataglanceseries.com/haematology

B₁₂ deficiency

Clinical features

- Gradual onset of features of anaemia.
- Mild jaundice, caused by ineffective erythropoiesis (Fig. 12.1).
- Glossitis and angular cheilosis and, if severe, sterility (either sex) and reversible melanin skin pigmentation.
- B_{12} deficiency causes a symmetrical neuropathy affecting the pyramidal tracts and posterior columns of the spinal cord (subacute combined degeneration of the cord) and the peripheral nerves. Patients present with tingling in the feet (more than the hands), difficulty in gait, visual or psychiatric disorders.
- B_{12} or folate deficiency in pregnancy is associated with increased incidence of fetal neural tube defects, e.g. spina bifida.
- Patients may be asymptomatic and detected by a routine blood test.

Laboratory findings

- Macrocytic anaemia with oval macrocytes and hypersegmented neutrophils (more than five nuclear lobes) (Fig. 12.2).
- Moderate reduction in leucocyte and platelet counts (severe cases).
- Biochemical tests in anaemic patients show raised serum bilirubin (indirect), lactate dehydrogenase.
- In B_{12} deficiency, the serum B_{12} is low, serum folate is normal or raised and red cell folate is normal or low.
- Bone marrow is hypercellular, increased proportion of early cells, megaloblastic erythropoiesis and giant metamyelocytes (Fig. 12.3).
- Raised serum methylmalonic acid (B_{12} deficiency), raised serum homocysteine (either B_{12} or folate deficiency).

Tests for causes of B₁₂ deficiency

These include history (diet, previous gastrointestinal surgery), tests for intrinsic factor (IF), antibody (positive in 50% of cases of PA) and parietal cell antibodies (positive in 90% of cases of PA), serum gastrin level (raised in PA) and upper gastrointestinal endoscopy.

Treatment

Treatment of B_{12} deficiency is 1 mg hydroxocobalamin intramuscularly, repeated every 2–3 days until six injections have been given; then one injection every 3 months for life unless the cause of deficiency has been corrected. Large doses of oral B_{12} can also be used.

Folate deficiency

The clinical features of folate deficiency are the same as B_{12} deficiency, but folate deficiency does not cause a similar neuropathy. Folic acid therapy in early pregnancy reduces the incidence of neural tube defects (NTD) (anencephaly, spina bifida, encephalocoele) in the fetus.

Tests for causes of folate deficiency

These include history (diet, previous surgery, drug therapy, alcohol, other associated diseases), transglutaminase and endomysial antibodies (positive in gluten-induced enteropathy), and other tests for malabsorption (e.g. duodenal biopsy). The serum folate is low, red cell folate low and serum B_{12} is normal or slightly reduced.

Treatment

Treatment is 5 mg folic acid daily for 4 months, then decide whether to continue folic acid, e.g. 5 mg folic acid once weekly or 400 μg daily indefinitely. Folate therapy corrects the anaemia but not the neuropathy of B_{12} deficiency. Indeed, administration of folic acid to a severely B_{12}-deficient individual may precipitate or worsen B_{12} neuropathy. Pregnant women are given folic acid 400 μg/day to reduce the incidence of megaloblastic anaemia and neural tube defects in the fetus. Dietary fortification with folate is used in the United States and 70 other countries (not the United Kingdom) to reduce the incidence of NTD.

Other causes of megaloblastic anaemia

Defects of B_{12} or folate metabolism include congenital transcobalamin (TC) II deficiency which leads to B_{12} malabsorption and failure of B_{12} to enter cells despite a normal (attached to TCI) serum B_{12} level. Megaloblastic anaemia (MA) occurs usually in early infancy. N_2O anaesthesia reversibly inactivates body B_{12}, and prolonged or repeated exposure may cause megaloblastic anaemia or B_{12} neuropathy. Antifolate drugs include the inhibitors of dihydrofolate reductase (methotrexate, pyrimethamine and trimethoprim) which have progressively less activity against the human compared to the bacterial enzyme. Folinic acid (5-formyl-THF) is used to overcome methotrexate or co-trimoxazole toxicity. Megaloblastic anaemia may occur with cytotoxic drug therapy (e.g. 6-mercaptopurine, cytosine arabinoside or hydroxycarbamide) or, rarely, because of inborn errors in DNA synthesis, e.g. orotic aciduria.

Causes of macrocytosis

Alcohol is the most frequent cause of large red cells. The haemoglobin level is usually normal. Mean corpuscular volume is not usually as high as in severe MA. White cell and platelet counts are normal in alcohol and the other conditions listed in Box 12.1, unless the underlying marrow disease affects these. Other distinguishing features from B_{12} or folate deficiency are that the red cells are circular rather than oval, hypersegmented neutrophils are absent and the marrow is normoblastic.

Box 12.1 Causes of raised mean corpuscular volume other than megaloblastic anaemia

1 Alcohol
2 Liver disease
3 Myxoedema
4 Reticulocytosis
5 Cytotoxic drugs
6 Aplastic anaemia
7 Pregnancy
8 Myelodysplastic syndromes
9 Myeloma
10 Neonatal

13.1 Red cell breakdown

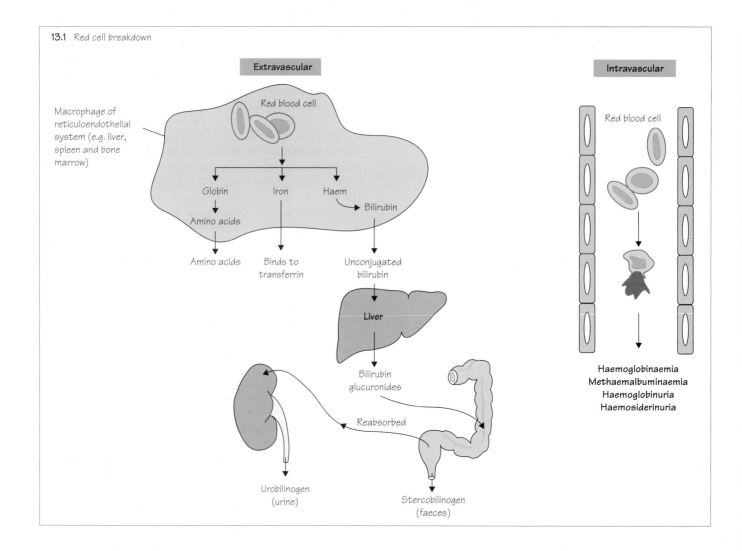

Haematology at a Glance, Fourth Edition. Atul B. Mehta and A. Victor Hoffbrand.

Haemolytic anaemias I: General

Haemolytic anaemias are caused by a shortened red cell lifespan; the normal mean red cell life (MRCL) is 120 days. Red cell production can be increased 6–8 times by normal bone marrow and haemolytic anaemia (HA) occurs if MRCL falls to 15 days or less, particularly in the presence of ineffective erythropoiesis, haematinic deficiency or marrow disease. Haemolysis may be caused by a fault in the red cell, usually inherited (Table 13.1), or an abnormality in its environment, usually acquired (Table 13.1).

Physiology of red cell destruction (Fig. 13.1)

Red cell destruction is normally extravascular in the macrophages of the reticuloendothelial system, e.g. in the bone marrow, liver and spleen. Globin is degraded to amino acids, haem to protoporphyrin, carbon monoxide and iron. Protoporphyrin is metabolized to bilirubin, conjugated to a glucuronide in the liver, excreted in faeces (as stercobilinogen) and, after reabsorption, in urine as urobilinogen.

Iron is recycled to plasma and combined to transferrin. Some iron remains in the macrophages as ferritin and haemosiderin. Haptoglobins are plasma proteins that bind haemoglobin to form a complex which is removed by the liver; their level is reduced in haemolysis as well as in liver disease. Pathological red cell destruction is also usually extravascular. However, it may be intravascular (Box 13.1). Some haemoglobin may then appear in plasma, where it is toxic and may cause fever, rigors and tissue damage. It is excreted unchanged in the urine and may cause renal damage. It is also partly reabsorbed by the renal tubules and broken down in the tubular cells to haemosiderin which appears in urine (Box 13.1).

Clinical features

- Anaemia (unless fully compensated haemolysis).
- Jaundice (usually mild) caused by unconjugated bilirubin in plasma; bilirubin is absent from the urine.
- An increased incidence of pigment (bilirubin) gallstones.
- Splenomegaly – in many types.
- Ankle ulcers, especially sickle cell anaemia, thalassaemia intermedia and hereditary spherocytosis.
- Expansion of marrow with, in children, bone expansion, e.g. frontal bossing in β-thalassaemia major.
- Aplastic crises caused by parvovirus infection.
- Megaloblastic anaemia caused by folate deficiency.

Laboratory features

Extravascular haemolysis
- Haemoglobin level may be normal or reduced.
- Raised reticulocyte count.
- Blood film may show polychromasia (blue staining in young red cells) and altered red cell shape, e.g. spherocytes, elliptocytes, sickle cells or fragmented cells.
- Bone marrow shows increased erythropoiesis.
- Serum indirect (unconjugated) bilirubin is raised.
- Serum haptoglobin absent.
- *Intravascular haemolysis* leads to raised plasma and urine haemoglobin, positive serum (Schumm) test for methaemalbumin, presence of haemosiderin in urine.

Table 13.1 Classification of haemolytic anaemia

Hereditary	Acquired
Membrane	**Immune**
Hereditary spherocytosis, hereditary elliptocytosis	*Autoimmune*
South-East Asian ovalocytosis	Warm antibody type
	Idiopathic or secondary to SLE, CLL, drugs, e.g. methyldopa
	Cold antibody type
	Idiopathic or secondary to infections (e.g. mycoplasma, infectious mononucleosis), lymphoma, paroxysmal cold haemoglobinuria
Metabolism	
G6PD deficiency	*Alloimmune*
Pyruvate kinase deficiency	Haemolytic transfusion reactions
Other rare enzyme deficiencies	Haemolytic disease of newborn
Haemoglobin	
Haemoglobin defect (Hb S, Hb C, unstable) (see Chapter 17)	**Red cell fragmentation syndromes**
	Cardiac valve, 'march' haemoglobinuria
	Microangiopathic haemolytic anaemia
	Thrombotic thrombocytopenia purpura
	Haemolytic uraemic syndrome
	Disseminated intravascular coagulation
	Infections
	e.g. malaria, clostridia
	Chemical and physical agents
	e.g. drugs, industrial/domestic substances, burns
	Secondary
	e.g. liver and renal disease
	Paroxysmal nocturnal haemoglobinuria

CLL, chronic lymphocytic leukaemia; SLE, systemic lupus erythematosus

---

Box 13.1 Causes of intravascular haemolysis

- Mismatched blood transfusion (usually ABO)
- G6PD deficiency with oxidant stress
- Red cell fragmentation syndromes
- Some autoimmune haemolytic anaemias
- Some drug- and infection-induced haemolytic anaemias
- Paroxysmal nocturnal haemoglobinuria
- March haemoglobinuria
- Unstable haemoglobin

Haemolytic anaemias II: inherited membrane and enzyme defects

14

14.1 Hereditary spherocytosis: peripheral blood film

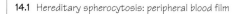

14.2 Hereditary spherocytosis: Flow cytometry showing reduced Eosin-5-maleimide staining in HS red cells

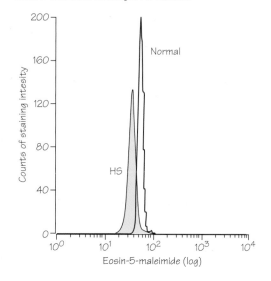

14.3 Glucose-6-phosphate dehydrogenase deficiency. Frequency in different geographical areas

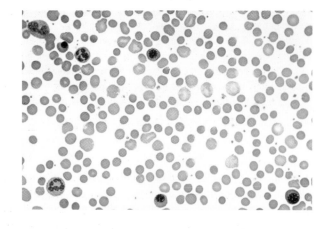

Lorenz von Seidelein et al. Malaria Journal, 2013, 12, 112 (with permission)

14.4 Glucose-6-phosphate dehydrogenase deficiency: peripheral blood film showing red cells which have 'blistered' cytoplasm, and where haemoglobin in cytoplasm is contracted and pulled away from the membrane to give a 'basket' cell

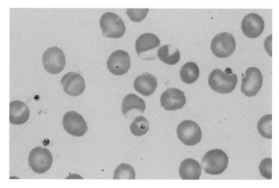

Membrane abnormalities

The normal red cell membrane consists of a lipid bipolar layer, vertical penetrating proteins and a horizontal protein skeleton consisting of α and β spectrin and proteins that join them to each other (Fig. 14.1).

Hereditary spherocytosis

This is the most common inherited haemolytic anaemia (HA) in white people. It is autosomal dominant with variable severity and may present as severe neonatal HA, as symptomatic HA later in life or may be an incidental finding. Defect is in a red cell membrane protein, e.g. ankyrin, band 3 or β-spectrin; 25% of cases are new mutations. Affected red cells lose membrane during passage through the reticuloendothelial system, especially the spleen. The cells become progressively more spherical (decreased surface area : volume ratio) and microcytic. They are destroyed prematurely, mainly in the spleen. Hereditary elliptocytosis (HE) is a similar, usually milder, abnormality, usually due to mutations of α or β spectrim.

Clinical features

Clinical features are those generally associated with HA. The spleen is usually enlarged.

Laboratory features

- Blood film: microspherocytes and polychromasia (Fig. 14.1).
- Haemoglobin level variable.
- Tests for HA are positive (see Chapter 13).
- Special test: Eosin-5-maleimide (EMA) test for band 3 abnormality usually positive (Fig. 14.2). This uses flow cytometry to determine the amount of fluorescence, affecting EMA binding to membrane proteins.
- Direct antiglobulin test is negative, excluding warm autoimmune HA which can cause a similar blood film appearance.

Treatment

- Splenectomy corrects the decrease in lifespan, although spherocytosis persists. Splenectomy may not be needed in mild cases; defer if possible in children until over the age of 6 years.
- Give folic acid prophylactically for severe cases.
- Pigment gallstones may cause cholecystitis.
- If cholecystectomy required, perform splenectomy also to reduce risk of recurrent gallstones.

South-East Asian ovalocytosis

This is an inherited red cell membrane protein defect (band 3), in which carriers have a degree of protection against malaria.

Enzyme abnormalities

Glucose-6-phosphate dehydrogenase deficiency

Glucose-6-phosphate dehydrogenase (G6PD) is the first enzyme in the hexose monophosphate pathway (see Fig. 2.7) which generates reducing power as reduced nicotinamide adenine dinucleotide phosphate (NADPH). Deficiency results in red cells being susceptible to oxidant stress. The gene is on the X chromosome so inheritance is sex linked. Males are typically affected, although females may show mild abnormalities. Many different DNA mutations within the gene give rise to mutant enzymes which are unstable and have reduced activity. Affected males develop HA when the red cells are exposed to oxidant stress, especially by drugs, infections, ingestion of fava beans and during the

---

Box 14.1 Agents that may cause haemolytic anaemia in G6PD deficiency

Infections and other acute illnesses, e.g. diabetic ketoacidosis
  Drugs
- Antimalarials, e.g. primaquine
- Sulfonamides and sulfones, e.g. co-trimoxazole, sulfanilamide, dapsone, salazopyrin
- Other antibacterial agents, e.g. nitrofurans, chloramphenicol
- Analgesics, e.g. aspirin (moderate doses are safe)
- Antihelminths, e.g. β-naphthol, stibophen, niridazole
- Miscellaneous, e.g. vitamin K analogues, naphthalene (mothballs), probenecid, rasburicase
  Fava beans (broad beans)

---

neonatal period (Box 14.1). Infection is associated with increased production of oxidants (e.g. H_2O_2) from neutrophils. G6PD deficiency is one of the most common of all inherited disorders and is common in black, Mediterranean, Middle Eastern and oriental populations (Fig. 14.3). Individuals with G6PD deficiency have a degree of protection against malaria.

Clinical and laboratory features

- Blood count and film normal between crises.
- During crises features of acute intravascular haemolysis; renal failure may occur in severe episodes.
- Blood film in a crisis shows red cells with absent haemoglobin ('bite' and 'blister' cells) and polychromasia (Fig. 14.4). Heinz bodies (denatured haemoglobin) may be seen in a reticulocyte preparation with supravital staining.
- Haemolysis is usually self-limited because of the increased G6PD activity in reticulocytes.
- Chronic non-spherocytic HA (CNSHA) occurs rarely with certain mutant enzymes.
- Neonatal jaundice is frequent.
- Screening tests for red cell G6PD deficiency measure the generation of NADPH. The enzyme may also be characterized by electrophoresis, assay of activity and DNA analysis. Diagnosis should, when possible, be undertaken in the steady state as reticulocytes generally have higher enzyme activity than mature red cells so the raised reticulocyte count following haemolysis may lead to a false normal result.

Management

- Stop offending drugs or fava bean ingestion.
- Treat infection if present.
- Transfuse red cells if necessary.
- Splenectomy may ameliorate HA in rare CNSHA.

Pyruvate kinase deficiency

Pyruvate kinase (PK) deficiency is the most frequent enzyme deficiency in the Embden–Meyerhof (glycolytic) pathway to cause CNSHA. Inheritance is autosomal recessive. The O_2-dissociation curve is shifted to the right, so symptoms are mild in comparison to the degree of anaemia. Splenectomy partly improves the anaemia.

Other enzyme deficiencies are rare causes of CNSHA and are frequently associated with musculoskeletal disease.

15.1 Warm autoimmune haemolytic anaemia: peripheral blood film. There is a circulating nucleated red blood cell (NRBC), polychromasia and microspherocytes

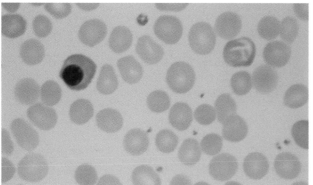

15.3 Thrombotic thrombocytopenic purpura (TTP): blood film showing red cell fragmentation with a circulating nucleated red blood cell and low platelet count

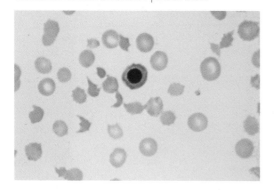

15.2 Direct antiglobulin (Coombs') test (DAT) is a means of detecting immunoglobulin and/or complement coating the red blood cells. Red blood cells are washed and anti-human globulin is added. This may be of broad specificity or specific, e.g. for IgG, IgA, IgM or complement. If agglutination occurs, then the red blood cells must have been coated; if no agglutination occurs, the red blood cells were not coated. In the indirect antiglobulin test, red cells are first incubated with serum at 37°C for 30 minutes a DAT is then performed, which will be positive if there are antibodies in the serum reacting against the red blood cells

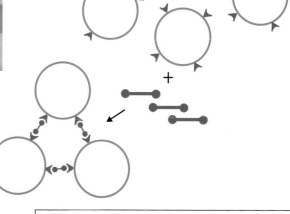

•—•	Anti-human globulin (AHG, Coombs' reagent)
◄	Antibody (IgG, IgM or IgA) or complement coating RBC
◯	Red blood cell

Autoimmune haemolytic anaemia

This is caused by autoantibodies against the red cell membrane. It is divided into warm and cold antibody types and each may be idiopathic or secondary to other diseases (see Table 13.1).

Warm autoimmune haemolytic anaemia

Antibody, typically IgG, has maximum activity at 37°C (Table 15.1).

Clinical and laboratory features

• Presents at any age, in either sex, with features of extravascular haemolytic anaemia of varying severity.
• The spleen is often enlarged.
• Blood film shows microspherocytes, polychromasia, ± circulating nucleated red blood cells (Fig. 15.1).
• Direct antiglobulin test (DAT) is positive (Fig. 15.2).
• Antibody may be non-specific or directed against antigens in the Rh system.
• IgG or IgG + complement (C3d) is detected on the red cell.
• Free antibody may be present in the serum.

Table 15.1 Autoimmune haemolytic anaemia. Comparison of warm and cold antibodies

	Warm	Cold
Class	IgG	IgM
Specificity	None or Rh	I (or i)
Optimal temperature of action	37°C	4°C
DAT	IgG or IgG + C3d	C3d
RBC destruction	Spleen or RES generally	RES generally
Associated diseases	CLL, SLE	Lymphoma, infectious mononucleosis

CLL, chronic lymphocytic leukaemia; DAT, direct antiglobulin test; Ig, immunoglobulin; RBC, red blood cell; RES, reticuloendothelial system; SLE, systemic lupus erythematosus.

- May be associated with immune thrombocytopenia (Evans' syndrome).
- Antibody-coated red cells are destroyed in the reticuloendothelial system, especially the spleen.

Treatment
- Corticosteroids, e.g. prednisolone 1 mg/kg orally with subsequent gradual reduction.
- Blood transfusion, if necessary.
- Other immunosuppressive drugs, e.g. rituximab (anti-CD20), azathioprine, ciclosporin, cyclophosphamide, mycophenolate.
- Consider splenectomy if steroid and other immunosuppressive drug therapy fails.
- Remove cause, e.g. drug.
- Treat underlying disease, e.g. chronic lymphocytic leukaemia, systemic lupus erythematosus.

Cold autoimmune haemolytic anaemia
Antibody, typically IgM, has maximum activity at 4°C.

Clinical and laboratory features
- Chronic haemolytic anaemia aggravated by cold. There may be acrocyanosis (purplish skin discoloration) or Raynaud phenomenon affecting the nose, ears, fingers and toes. Haemolysis may be intravascular and if severe may cause rigors, haemoglobinuria, renal failure.
- Positive DAT with C3d on red cells.
- Cold agglutinins, usually IgM and directed against I (or i antigen especially in infectious mononucleosis) on red cells, are present in serum, often to titres of 1:4000 or more. In primary form (cold haemagglutinin disease), the antibody is monoclonal and the patient may ultimately develop non-Hodgkin lymphoma.
- Paroxysmal cold haemoglobinuria is a rare syndrome, precipitated by infections. Intravascular haemolysis is caused by the Donath–Landsteiner antibody which binds red cells in the cold, but causes lysis at 37°C.

Treatment
- Keep the patient warm.
- Consider immunosuppression with chlorambucil, cyclophosphamide, fludarabine, rituximab.
- Consider plasma exchange to lower antibody titre.

Alloimmune haemolytic anaemia
This is caused when antibody produced by one individual reacts against red cells of another. The three important situations are:
1 Mismatched blood transfusion (see Chapter 49);
2 Haemolytic disease of the newborn (see Chapter 47); and
3 Following marrow or solid organ transplantation.

Drug-induced immune haemolytic anaemia
These include: (a) an antibody against a drug-red cell membrane complex (e.g. penicillin), (b) deposition of an immune complex of drug and plasma protein on the red cell surface, or (c) stimulation of an autoantibody, e.g. methydopa.

Red cell fragmentation syndromes
These occur when red cells are exposed to an abnormal surface (e.g. non-endothelialized artificial heart valve), cardiac haemolytic anaemia or flow through small vessels containing fibrin strands (e.g. in disseminated intravascular coagulation) or damaged small vessels (microangiopathic haemolytic anaemia; MAHA). This occurs in thrombotic thrombocytopenic purpura, haemolytic uraemic syndrome, widespread adenocarcinoma, malignant hypertension, pre-eclampsia and meningococcal septicaemia. Haemolysis is both extravascular and intravascular; blood film shows deeply staining fragmented red cells (Fig. 15.3). Serum lactate dehydrogenase (LDG) is raised.

Infections
These may cause haemolysis by:
- Direct damage to red cells (e.g. malaria);
- Toxin production (e.g. *Clostridium perfringens*);
- Oxidant stress in G6PD-deficient individuals;
- MAHA (e.g. meningococcal septicaemia);
- Autoantibody formation (e.g. infectious mononucleosis) and
- Extravascular destruction (e.g. malaria).

Chemical and physical agents
Some drugs, e.g. dapsone, or chemicals, e.g. chlorate, cause haemolysis by oxidation even with normal G6PD levels. Severe burns and snakebites may also cause haemolysis.

Paroxysmal nocturnal haemoglobinuria
This is a clonal disorder in which haemolysis is caused by a rare acquired mutation of the *PIG-A* gene in haemopoietic stem cells. This results in a defect of the phosphatidyl inositol anchor which tethers a large number of proteins to the cell membrane. The cells become abnormally sensitive to complement-mediated haemolysis because of lack of proteins that protect against complement, e.g. CD55 (DAF) and CD59 (MIRL). It is often associated with a hypoplastic marrow with neutropenia and thrombocytopenia. The clinical course is frequently complicated by recurrent venous thromboses, especially of large veins, e.g. hepatic or portal; also by iron deficiency and infections. Diagnosis is made by the presence of red cells or white cells lacking the CD55 or CD59 antigens.

Treatment
Iron is given for iron deficiency resulting from chronic intravascular haemolysis.
- Transfusion of leucodepleted red cells may be necessary.
- Warfarin may be needed lifelong to prevent thrombosis.
- A monoclonal antibody, Eculizumab, which inhibits the activation of terminal complement components by binding to C5, is used to reduce haemolysis, thrombosis, and improve life expectancy.
- Allogeneic stem cell transplant is considered for serious cases in young adults.

16 Haemolytic anaemias IV: genetic defects of haemoglobin – thalassaemia

16.1 The globin genes are located on chromosomes 16 (ζ, α) and 11 (ε, γ, δ, β). A 5' locus control region (LCR) is important in regulating γ and β globin gene expression. Different genes are transcribed during pre- and postnatal life, and the chains are synthesized independently and then combine to produce the different haemoglobins. The γ genes differ to produce either a glutamic acid (Gγ) or alanine (Aγ) residue at position 136. Whereas haemopoiesis occurs in yolk sac, liver and spleen prenatally, it is confined to marrow postnatally

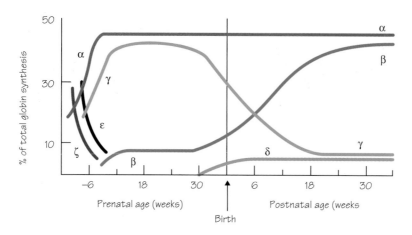

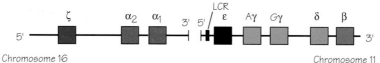

16.2 The ratio of α to β globin synthesis in α and β thalassaemia syndromes.
βO = absent β gene function; β+ = reduced β gene function

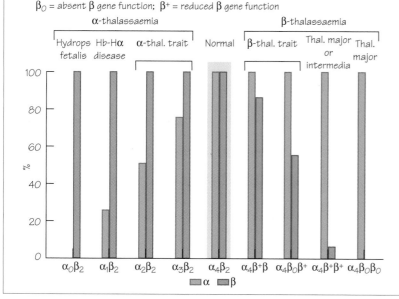

16.3 β-Thalassaemia major: skull X-ray showing expansion of the medullary cavity giving rise to a 'hair on end' appearance

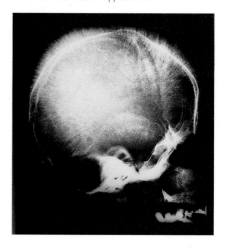

Haematology at a Glance, Fourth Edition. Atul B. Mehta and A. Victor Hoffbrand.

16.4 β-Thalassaemia major: peripheral blood film showing hypochromic microcytic red cells, target cells, poikilocytes and nucleated red blood cells. The few well-haemoglobinized cells are transfused red cells

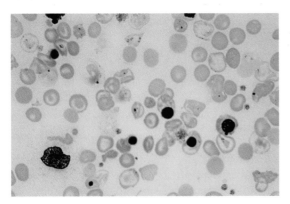

16.6 Cellulose acetate eletrophoresis of haemoglobin; normal (A+A) and carriers for haemoglobin C, haemoglobin S or both S and C

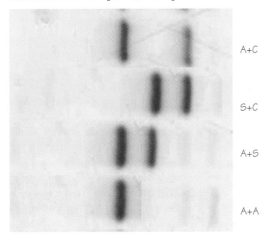

A+C

S+C

A+S

A+A

16.5 High performance liquid chromatography.
(a) HPLC printout showing a patient with β-thalassaemia trait – major band of HbA with increased concentrations of HbA2 and HbF.
(b) A patient with sickle cell trait and two bands corresponding to HbA and HbS

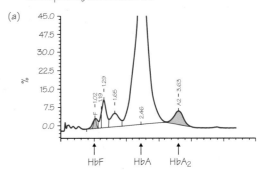

(a)

HbF   HbA   HbA₂

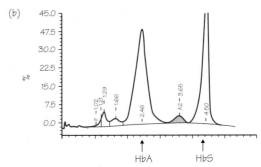

(b)

HbA   HbS

Normal haemoglobins

The haemoglobins are made up of four globin chains each containing a haem group. Embryonic haemoglobins (Portland, Gower I and II) are present in early fetal life. Fetal haemoglobin (Hb F, $\alpha_2\gamma_2$) dominates by late fetal life. Hb F has a higher oxygen affinity than Hb A and this allows the fetus to obtain oxygen from the mother (Fig. 2.3). A switch occurs at 3–6 months in the neonatal period to normal adult haemoglobin (Hb A, $\alpha_2\delta_2$) (Fig. 16.1). Low levels of Hb F and the minor adult haemoglobin Hb A_2 ($\alpha_2\delta_2$) are also present in normal adults (see Table 2.1).

Genetic disorders of haemoglobin

1 Disorders of α- or β-globin chain synthesis (the thalassaemias) (Table 16.1; Fig. 16.2);
2 Structural defects of haemoglobin which give rise to haemolysis (e.g. sickle cell anaemia, haemoglobin C);
3 Unstable haemoglobins (rare); and
4 Structural disorders giving rise to polycythaemia or methaemoglobinaemia (rare).

The first and second have a wide global prevalence, particularly where malaria is, or was, common, as the carrier states give some protection against falciparum malaria. Compound heterozygote states of a thalassaemic allele and a haemoglobin structural variant allele frequently occur and include sickle/β-thalassaemia and Hb E/β-thalassaemia.

Thalassaemia

These autosomal recessive syndromes divide into α- and β-thalassaemia depending on whether there is reduced synthesis of α- or β-globin (Table 16.1, Fig. 16.2).

α-Thalassaemia

Normally there are four α-globin genes, two on each chromosome 16 (Fig. 16.1). The severity of α-thalassaemia depends on the number of α-genes deleted or, less frequently, dysfunctional.

Hydrops foetalis

If all four α-genes are inactive hydrops foetalis occurs. The fetus is unable to make either fetal ($\alpha_2\gamma_2$) or adult Hb A ($\alpha_2\beta_2$) haemoglobin. Death occurs *in utero* or neonatally.

Table 16.1 Classification of thalassaemia

Clinical phenotype	Thalassaemia (thal) syndrome
Hydrops foetalis	Homozygous α-thal major → complete lack of α-globin
Thalassaemia major	Homozygous β or doubly heterozygous β thal → complete or almost complete lack of β-globin
Thalassaemia intermedia	See below
Thalassaemia trait	Heterozygous β-thalassaemia (β-thal minor, lack of one functional β-globin gene[*]) Heterozygous α-thalassaemia (α-thal minor, lack of one or two α-globin genes[†])

[*]Normal individual has two (one from each parent on each allele)
[†]Normal individual has four (two from each parent on each allele)

Haemoglobin H disease

This is caused by deletion or functional inactivity of three of the four α-genes. Markedly microcytic, hypochromic anaemia (Hb 60–110 g/L) with splenomegaly is usual. Bone deformities and features of iron overload usually do not occur. Haemoglobin electrophoresis shows 4–10% haemoglobin H (β_4) and supravital staining shows 'golf ball' cells.

α-Thalassaemia trait

This is caused by deletion or dysfunction of one or two α-genes. It is characterized by microcytic, hypochromic red cells with a raised red cell count ($>5.5 \times 10^9$/L). Mild anaemia occurs in some cases with two α-genes deleted.

β-Thalassaemia

Thalassaemia major

Complete ($\beta^0\beta^0$) or almost complete ($\beta^0\beta^+$) failure of β-globin chain synthesis resulting from inheritance from each parent of one of over 400 different point mutations or deletions in the β-globin gene or its controlling sequences. There is a severe imbalance of $\alpha:\beta$-chains (Fig. 16.2) with deposition of α-chains in erythroblasts, ineffective erythropoiesis, severe anaemia and extramedullary haemopoiesis.

Clinical features

- Anaemia presents at the age of 3–6 months when the switch from γ- to β-chain synthesis normally occurs. Milder cases present later (up to the age of 4 years).
- Failure to thrive, intercurrent infection, pallor, mild jaundice.
- Enlargement of the liver and spleen, expansion of the bones resulting from bone marrow hyperplasia – especially of the skull – with bossing and a 'hair-on-end' appearance on X-ray (Fig. 16.3); thalassaemic facies, caused by expansion of skull and facial bones.
- Features of iron overload as a result of blood transfusions and increased iron absorption include melanin pigmentation, growth/endocrine defects, e.g. diabetes mellitus, hypothyroidism, hypoparathyroidism, failure of sexual development, cardiac failure or arrhythmia, liver abnormality (see Chapter 10).

Laboratory findings

- Severe anaemia (Hb 20–60 g/L) with reduced mean corpuscular volume and mean corpuscular haemoglobin.
- Blood film (Fig. 16.4) shows hypochromic, microcytic cells, target cells, erythroblasts and, often, myelocytes.
- Bone marrow is hypercellular with erythroid hyperplasia.
- High performance liquid chromatography (Fig. 16.5) or haemoglobin electrophoresis (Fig. 16.6) can be used to measure the concentration of the different haemoglobins present in red cells. No haemoglobin A is detected in $\beta^0\beta^0$ patients.
- DNA analysis reveals the specific mutations or deletions.

Management

- Regular transfusions of packed red cells to maintain haemoglobin above 90–100 g/L, leucodepleted to reduce risk of human leucocyte antigen (HLA) sensitization and transmission of disease, e.g. cytomegalovirus.
- Iron chelation therapy has been with subcutaneous desferrioxamine (DFO) over 8–12 hours on 5–7 nights weekly. This produces both urinary and faecal excretion of iron. Oral vitamin C increases iron excretion with DFO. Side effects of DFO include hearing loss, visual

defects, bone and cartilage defects and growth impairment. The main problem with its use is lack of compliance and the presence of cardiac iron overload even in some patients complying with the treatment.

Two orally active iron chelators are now available. Deferiprone (DFP) is given in three daily doses and is more effective than DFO at removing cardiac iron. It causes urinary excretion of iron: side effects include neutropenia, agranulocytosis (1% of patients), gastrointestinal disturbances and arthralgia. Deferasirox (DFX) causes increased loss of iron in faeces. It is given once daily, may cause skin rashes, gastrointestinal and renal toxicity but is generally well tolerated. Its cardioprotective effectiveness remains to be fully established. Combination of chelators may be more effective than single drug therapy. DFO and deferiprone given simultaneously cause additive or even synergistic iron secretion with excellent clinical results. This combination is used for patients in iron-induced heart failure.

Iron chelation therapy is monitored clinically and by changes in serum ferritin by cardiac and liver function and cardiac iron measured by T2* MRI. The cardiac T2* value can predict which patients are likely to develop cardiac failure or arrhythmia.

• Hepatitis B is prevented by early immunization. Patients who already have chronic active hepatitis caused by hepatitis C may need α-interferon + ribavirin and new antihepatitis C drug therapy.

• Splenectomy is necessary if blood requirements are excessively high. Defer if possible until the age of 5 years, precede by immunization against capsulated organisms (see Chapter 19) and follow by oral penicillin therapy for life. If the platelet count remains raised, low-dose aspirin reduces the risk of thromboembolism.

• Stem cell transplantation from an HLA-matching sibling may give long-term disease-free survival of up to 90% in good-risk patients, but nearer 50% in poor risk (previously poorly chelated with iron overload and liver fibrosis).

• Treat complications of iron overload: heart, endocrine organs, liver damage.

• Osteoporosis may occur as a result of marrow expansion, endocrine deficiencies. It is treated with calcium, vitamin D and, if needed, bisphosphonate therapy.

Thalassaemia intermedia

This is a variable syndrome milder than thalassaemia major, with later onset, and characterized by moderately severe (Hb 60–100 g/L), hypochromic, microcytic anaemia requiring either few or no transfusions. There is milder imbalance of $\alpha : \beta + \gamma$-globin chain synthesis than in thalassaemia major. This may be because of inheritance of a milder β-chain defect, increased capacity to produce γ-chains or co-inheritance of β-chain defects with an α-thalassaemia allele leading to reduced $\alpha : \beta$ chain imbalance. Hepatosplenomegaly, extramedullary haemopoiesis, anaemia and bone deformities may occur. Iron overload increases with age as a result of irregular blood transfusions and increased gastrointestinal iron absorption. Iron chelation therapy may be needed.

β-Thalassaemia trait

This is a mild hypochromic, microcytic anaemia with a raised red cell count ($>5.5 \times 10^{12}$/L) and raised haemoglobin A$_2$ ($\alpha_2\delta_2$) level ($>3.5\%$). Iron stores are normal. Accurate diagnosis allows genetic counselling and avoidance of inappropriate iron therapy.

Prenatal diagnosis of haemoglobin defects

Prenatal diagnosis is available using DNA (chorionic villous or amniotic fluid). Carriers must first be identified (screening by blood count in ethnic minority groups, at preconception counselling or in the antenatal clinic). If a mother is a carrier, her partner must be tested. If both are carriers, there is a one in four chance that the fetus is homozygous (or doubly heterozygous) or normal and a one in two chance that it is a carrier. Fetal DNA is usually amplified by use of the polymerase chain reaction and the DNA mutations are detected. If the fetus is severely affected, e.g. by thalassaemia major, the couple should be counselled and termination of pregnancy offered, if appropriate.

17 Haemolytic anaemias V: genetic defects of haemoglobin – sickle cell disease

17.1 Effect of deoxygenation on red cells containing HbS ($\alpha_2\beta_{S2}$)

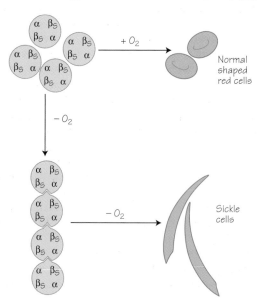

Normal shaped red cells

Sickle cells

17.2 Blood film in sickle cell disease showing a sickle cell (A), a target cell (B) and a red cell with a Howell-Jolly body (HJB) (C). HJBs are removed by spleen; adult patients with sickle cell disease have reduced spleen function

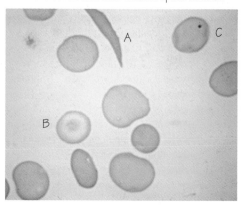

17.3 Sickle cell anaemia: bony changes. X-ray showing avascular necrosis of the head of the humerus

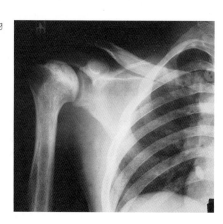

Sickle cell disease

Sickle cell disease (homozygous sickle cell anaemia) is a chronic haemolytic anaemia caused by a point mutation in the β-globin gene resulting in substitution of valine for glutamic acid in the sixth position of the β-globin chain. This causes insolubility of Hb S in its deoxygenated state. The insoluble chains crystallize in the red cells causing sickling (Fig. 17.1) and vascular occlusion. The disease is most common in Africans (one in five West Africans are carriers – they have some protection against falciparum malaria). The mutant gene also occurs in other parts of the world where malaria is, or was, prevalent, e.g. the Middle East, Far East and the Indian subcontinent.

Clinical features

These resemble those of other chronic haemolytic anaemias, punctuated with different types of crisis.

1 Vaso-occlusive crisis is caused by increased sickling with blockage of small vessels. Common precipitants are infection, dehydration, acidosis and deoxygenation. Abdominal pain is caused by infarction

Haematology at a Glance, Fourth Edition. Atul B. Mehta and A. Victor Hoffbrand.

affecting abdominal organs; bone pain may occur in the back, pelvis, ribs and long bones (Fig. 17.3). Infarction may affect the central nervous system – causing a stroke or fits – the lungs, spleen or kidneys. In children, the 'hand-foot syndrome' is caused by infarction of the metaphyses of the small bones.

2 Visceral sequestration crisis is caused by sickling with pooling of red cells in the liver, spleen or lungs. Sequestration in the lungs is partly responsible for the acute chest syndrome, though infarction and infection contribute.

3 Aplastic crisis occurs following infection by B19 parvovirus. This causes temporary arrest of erythropoiesis which in healthy individuals is of no consequence, but in patients with reduced red cell survival, such as Hb SS, can rapidly cause severe anaemia requiring blood transfusion. Folate deficiency due to increased utilization combined with poor diet may also cause anaemia.

Other clinical features

• Increased susceptibility to infection. Splenic function is reduced because infarction leads to autosplenectomy. Pneumococcal infections may lead to pneumonia and meningitis. Infarction of intestinal mucosa predisposes to *Salmonella* infection and osteomyelitis may result.

• Clinical features include pigment gallstones with cholecystitis, chronic leg ulcers, avascular necrosis of the femoral and humeral heads (Fig. 17.2) or other bones (due to repeated vaso-occlusive crises), cardiomyopathy, pulmonary hypertension, proliferative retinopathy, priapism and renal papillary necrosis (leading to polyuria, failure to concentrate urine and tendency to dehydration).

• Cranial Doppler studies can reveal abnormal blood flow due to stenosis predisposing to stroke. It is needed in all children older than 2 years. Retinal examination annually is performed after the age of 10 years.

Laboratory features

• Haemoglobin level is 70–90 g/L, but symptoms of anaemia are usually mild (the O_2 dissociation curve of Hb S is shifted to the right, see Chapter 2).

• Blood film shows sickle cells, and unusually target cells and often features of splenic atrophy (Fig. 17.2).

• Screening tests for sickling demonstrate increased turbidity of the blood after deoxygenation (e.g. with dithionate or Na_2HPO_4). Haemoglobin electrophoresis or high-performance liquid chromatography (Fig. 16.5, 16.6) shows haemoglobin with an abnormal migration. In Hb SS, there is absence of Hb A. Hb F level is usually mildly raised (5–10%).

Treatment

• General – avoid known precipitants of sickle cell crisis, especially dehydration and infections. Give pneumococcal, *Haemophilus influenzae* type B and meningococcal vaccination, and oral penicillin indefinitely to compensate for splenic atrophy.

• Folic acid is given to prevent folate deficiency.

• Fever in children with sickle cell disease needs urgent attention. Blood count, blood and urine culture and chest X-ray are performed and a lumbar puncture if meningitis is suspected. Very young children or older children with sepsis should be admitted to hospital for intravenous antibiotic therapy.

• Vaso-occlusive crisis is treated with hydration, usually intravenous normal saline; analgesia (e.g. diamorphine subcutaneous infusion); O_2 if there is hypoxia; antibiotics if there is infection.

• Red cell transfusion for severe anaemia (sequestration or aplastic crisis) or as a 3–12-month programme of therapy for patients with frequently recurring crises or for 2–3 years following central nervous system crisis, or for patients in whom Doppler studies predict for stroke.

• Severe sickling or sequestration crisis (e.g. 'chest syndrome' and stroke) is treated acutely with exchange transfusion to reduce Hb S levels to <30%. Pregnant patients and those undergoing general anaesthesia may need transfusion to reduce Hb S levels to <30%.

• Oral hydroxycarbamide (20–40 mg/kg/day) reduces both the frequency and duration of sickle cell crises. Although its precise mode of action is not known, it increases Hb F production, decreases intracellular Hb S concentration by increasing mean corpuscular volume, lowers the neutrophil count and inhibits prothrombotic interactions between sickle cells and the endothelium. It is widely used both in adults and in children.

• Stem cell transplantation in selected cases. The cure rate is about 85% in children younger than 16 years.

• Joint replacement surgery may be required for avascular necrosis (hips and shoulder).

• Iron chelation therapy for patients with iron overload caused by multiple transfusions (see Chapter 10).

Sickle cell trait

Sickle cell trait is a benign condition without anaemia and is usually asymptomatic. Occasionally, haematuria or overt crisis in conditions of oxygen deprivation, e.g. high mountains, occurs. Genetic counselling should be offered to carriers.

Other sickling disorders

Hb S may occur in combination with other genetic defects of haemoglobin (compound heterozygotes). Hb S/β-thalassaemia clinically resembles Hb SS but the spleen usually remains enlarged and mean corpuscular volume is reduced. Hb SC disease varies in severity from mild to indistinguishable from sickle cell anaemia; thrombotic complications and a proliferative retinopathy are particularly common.

Other structural haemoglobin abnormalities

Many other mutations of the α- or β-chain genes have been identified. Most that have a significant population frequency (e.g. Hb D) are not associated with clinical symptoms. However, some, e.g. Hb E, common in the Far East, may cause significant anaemia in a homozygous state or if co-inherited with a β-thalassaemia allele. Haemoglobin C, frequent in West Africa, causes a mild haemolytic anaemia in the homozygous state.

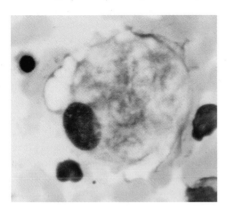

18.1 Histiocyte laden with glucocerebroside showing a fibrillar cytoplasmic pattern (Gaucher cell)

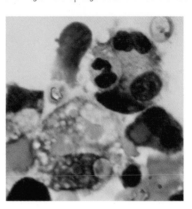

18.2 Haemophagocytic syndrome: bone marrow aspirate showing a macrophage laden with cellular debris

The common benign disorders of white cells arise as a response to a systemic process, e.g. infection, inflammation or malignancy.

Granulocytes and monocytes

An increased number of neutrophils in peripheral blood (neutrophil leucocytosis or neutrophilia) is most commonly due to bacterial infection or other causes of inflammation (Box 18.1).

In bacterial infection, neutrophil granules may stain intensely (toxic granulation) and Döhle bodies (cytoplasmic RNA) may be present. Corticosteroid therapy is also a common cause of neutrophilia. A leukaemoid reaction is a profound reactive neutrophilia in which granulocyte precursors (e.g. myelocytes) appear in the blood.

Neutropenia (reduced number of circulating neutrophils; Box 18.2) is usually due to decreased marrow production. Neutropenia can occur rarely in overwhelming bacterial infection, e.g. septicaemia, bacterial endocarditis. It increases susceptibility to infection, particularly bacterial. Viral infections are a common cause of neutropenia. Chemotherapy or radiotherapy are other frequent causes of neutropenia, which may be severe and life-threatening. The normal neutrophil count is lower in Afro-Caribbean and Middle Eastern subjects than in white people; this has no clinical consequences.

Causes of **eosinophilia** are listed in Box 18.3. Eosinophilia can occur in response to a range of systemic conditions including parasitic infection, certain malignancies (particularly Hodgkin lymphoma), allergy and connective tissue disease. **Basophilia** (increase in blood basophils to >0.1 × 10^9/L) is uncommon but occurs in myeloproliferative disorders. **Monocytosis** (increase in circulating monocytes to >1.0 × 10^9/L) may occur in chronic infections (bacterial and protozoal, particularly in patients who cannot mount a neutrophil response), in malignancy and in myelodysplasia (see Chapter 25).

Disorders of neutrophil function may be congenital or acquired and affect neutrophil interaction with immunoglobulin/complement, migration, phagocytosis and microbicidal activity. *Chronic granulo-*

Box 18.1 Causes of neutrophilia (neutrophils >7.5 × 10^9/L)

Reactive
- Bacterial infections
- Inflammation, e.g. collagen diseases, Crohn's disease
- Trauma and/or surgery
- Tissue necrosis/infarction
- Neoplasia
- Haemorrhage and haemolysis
- Metabolic, e.g. diabetic ketoacidosis
- Pregnancy

Malignant
- Myeloproliferative disorders
- Myeloid leukaemias

Drugs
- Steroids
- Granulocyte colony-stimulating factor (GCSF)

matous disease is a rare inherited (X-linked) condition in which neutrophils are able to phagocytose but not kill. Acquired defects occur, for example, in diabetes, myelodysplasia and corticosteroid therapy.

Lysosomal storage disease

Hereditary deficiencies of enzymes required for glycolipid metabolism lead to the accumulation of incompletely degraded macromolecules in various cells and tissues. *Gaucher disease* is the most common (autosomal recessive) and is caused by mutations in the gene encoding glucocerebrosidase A *(GBA)*. Type I (most common) occurs especially among Ashkenazi Jews (age of presentation from infancy to middle

age) and does not involve the central nervous system (CNS); types II
and III are rarer and do involve the CNS. Clinical features (enlarged
liver and spleen, characteristic bone defects) and haematological features (anaemia, thrombocytopenia with easy bruising) result from
accumulation of Gaucher cells (Fig. 18.1) in the spleen, liver, skeleton,
marrow and in types II and III in the CNS. Treatment is principally
by enzyme replacement therapy which is given by intravenous infusion. Oral treatments, which work by reducing the production of the
undegraded material, are increasingly used.

Histiocyte disorders

Histiocytes are the terminally differentiated cells of the monocyte–
macrophage system and are widely distributed throughout all tissues.
Langerhans cells are macrophages present in epidermis, spleen,
thymus, bone, lymph nodes and mucosal surfaces. *Langerhans cell
histiocytosis* (LCH) is a rare single organ or system or multisystem
disease occurring principally in childhood (<10 years), with an incidence of two to three cases per million population. Clinical features
include skin rash, bone pain/swelling, lymphadenopathy, hepatosplenomegaly, endocrine changes (e.g. diabetes insipidus as a result
of posterior pituitary involvement) and skeletal lesions. Malignant
histiocyte disorders include monocytic variants of acute leukaemia
(see Chapters 22 and 23) and some types of non-Hodgkin lymphoma
(see Chapter 34).

Haemophagocytic syndromes

In these syndromes, the bone marrow shows increased numbers of
histiocytes which contain ingested blood cells, leading to pancytopenia. The mechanism is poorly understood and prognosis is usually
poor. Causes include infection (viral, bacterial, tuberculosis), especially in an immunosuppressed host, tumours (e.g. lymphoma; Fig.
18.2) or rare familial types.

19.1 Peripheral blood lymphocytes (activated T cells) in infectious mononucleosis

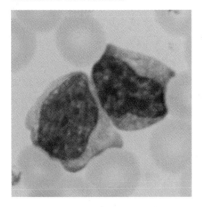

19.3 MRI scan of brain in a person with HIV. A mass is present, pressing on the third ventricle. Biopsy showed a high grade lymphoma

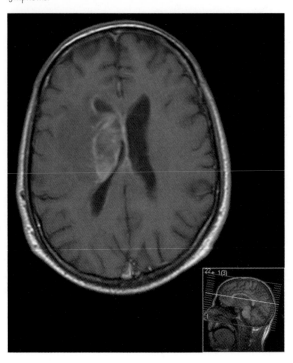

19.2 Screening test for infectious mononucleosis (IM). In the monospot slide test a drop of patient serum is added to red cell particles sensitized with a bovine mononucleosis antigen. The red cells agglutinate if the patients' serum contains anti-bovine antibody

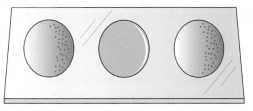

| Positive control | Negative control | Patient sample Result: POSITIVE |

Lymphocytosis occurs in viral infections, some bacterial infections (e.g. pertussis) and in lymphoid neoplasia. *Lymphopenia* (reduction in circulating lymphocytes to $<1.5 \times 10^9$/L) occurs in viral infection (e.g. HIV), lymphoma, connective tissue disease, severe bone marrow failure and with immunosuppressive drug therapy. Lymphadenopathy is lymph node enlargement, which may be local or generalized. Causes are listed in Box 19.1.

Infectious mononucleosis (*glandular fever*) is caused by Epstein–Barr virus (EBV) infection of B lymphocytes. Atypical circulating lymphocytes are reactive T cells. Cytomegalovirus, other viruses and *Toxoplasma* infections cause a similar blood picture (Fig. 19.1). Clinical features include onset usually in young adults (age 15–40 years), sore throat, lymphadenopathy, fever, morbilliform rash – particularly following treatment with amoxicillin – and jaundice, hepatomegaly and tender splenomegaly in a minority. Complications include autoimmune thrombocytopenia and/or haemolytic anaemia, myocarditis, neuropathy, encephalitis, hepatitis and postviral fatigue syndrome. The Paul–Bunnell test, modified as the monospot slide test (Fig. 19.2), detects heterophile antibodies (antibodies against cells of a different species). These agglutinate sheep or ox (bovine) red blood cells. The test is positive from 1 week after infection and persists for up to 2 months. Viral culture from sputum/saliva and specific IgM and IgG antibody tests against EBV nuclear and capsular antigens are sometimes useful in diagnosis.

Immunodeficiency

Depressed humoral immunity may be congenital (e.g. X-linked agammaglobulinaemia) or acquired (e.g. myeloma and chronic lymphocytic leukaemia; CLL) and characteristically leads to recurrent pyogenic bacterial infections. Depressed cell-mediated immunity may be congenital (e.g. DiGeorge syndrome) or acquired (e.g. HIV infection, lymphoma, CLL) and causes susceptibility to viral, protozoal and fungal infections, anergy and a secondary defect in humoral immunity. Mixed B- and T-cell deficiency is common.

Hyposplenism

Impaired splenic function or splenectomy reduces the body's ability to make antibody (particularly to capsulated organisms, e.g. pneumococcus, *Haemophilus*, meningococcus), reduces clearance of intracellular organisms (e.g. parasitized red cells) and impairs defence against organisms and toxins in the portal circulation. Splenic function may be impaired as a result of congenital absence of the spleen. Acquired

Box 19.1 Causes of lymphadenopathy

Local

Localized bacterial/viral infection

Skin condition, e.g. trauma, eczema

Malignant – secondary carcinoma, lymphoma

General

Infection:
- Bacterial, e.g. endocarditis, tuberculosis
- Viral, e.g. HIV, infectious mononucleosis, cytomegalovirus
- Other, e.g. toxoplasmosis, malaria

Malignancy

  e.g. lymphoma, lymphoid leukaemias

Inflammatory disorders

  e.g. sarcoidosis, connective tissue diseases

Generalized allergic conditions

  e.g. widespread eczema

Box 19.2 Causes of splenomegaly

Haemolytic anaemia

Hereditary spherocytosis, autoimmune haemolytic anaemia, thalassaemia major or intermedia, sickle cell anaemia (before infarction occurs)

Haematological malignancies

Lymphoma, CLL, ALL, AML, CML*

Polycythaemia vera, chronic myelofibrosis*

Myelodysplasia

Storage diseases

Gaucher disease*

Amyloid

Liver disease and portal hypertension
Congestive cardiac failure
Infection

Malaria*

Leishmaniasis*

Bacterial endocarditis

Viral infections, e.g. infectious mononucleosis

ALL, acute lymphoblastic leukaemia; AML, acute myeloid leukaemia; CLL, chronic lymphocytic leukaemia; CML, chronic myeloid leukaemia
*Causes of massive splenomegaly

hyposplenism occurs when there is recurrent thrombosis affecting the arterial systemic blood flow to the spleen (e.g. sickle cell disease, essential thrombocythaemia), infiltration of the spleen (e.g. amyloid), in gluten-induced enteropathy and, less frequently, inflammatory bowel disease or in the presence of high levels of circulating immune complexes (e.g. autoimmune diseases).

Splenomegaly

An enlarged spleen is often symptomless but may cause abdominal discomfort. It may cause pancytopenia (hypersplenism) with anaemia also due to dilution (increased plasma volume). Causes of an enlarged spleen are listed in Box 19.2. Inflammation and infection typically cause an increase in the white cell areas (white pulp), while congestion causes an increase in the red cell areas (red pulp). Proliferation of malignant cells, infiltration, storage disease and extramedullary haemopoiesis are other causes of enlargement.

Splenectomy

Splenectomy is beneficial in a number of haematological conditions, particularly when the spleen is the site of excessive destruction of peripheral blood cells, e.g. selected patients with haemolytic anaemia and thrombocytopenia (particularly autoimmune), and myelofibrosis. The spleen has an important role in removing capsulated and opsonized bacteria (see Chapter 3), and splenectomy (or hyposplenism due to disease, see above) leads to an increased susceptibility to infection. The operation should be avoided in children below 5 years and should be preceded by vaccination against pneumococcus, *Haemophilus influenzae* type B and meningococcus. Patients who are hyposplenic or post-splenectomy should take a prophylactic antibiotic indefinitely (e.g. oral penicillin V or erythromycin at low dose) and should carry a card at all times informing of their condition. Malaria is also likely to be more severe.

HIV infection and AIDS

HIV-1 is a retrovirus transmitted by semen, blood and other body fluids, which infects and kills CD4+ T lymphocytes to cause immune suppression. A non-specific febrile illness with lymphadenopathy often marks initial infection. A proportion of patients progress to AIDS with a CD4 count $<0.2 \times 10^9$/L. Clinical manifestations include recurring infections, anaemia and lymphadenopathy. There is an increased risk of non-Hodgkin lymphoma (especially high grade and involving the CNS; Fig. 19.3), Kaposi sarcoma and other tumours, e.g. Hodgkin lymphoma, acute myeloid leukaemia. Treatment may also induce anaemia; e.g. both azidothymidine (AZT) and co-trimoxazole cause megaloblastic change. Thrombocytopenia, lymphopenia and neutropenia (immune or caused by marrow failure or drug therapy) are also frequent. The bone marrow is usually normo- or hypercellular, with dysplastic features and an increase in plasma cells. A serum paraprotein occurs in 10–15% of cases.

20 Introduction to haematological malignancy: basic mechanisms

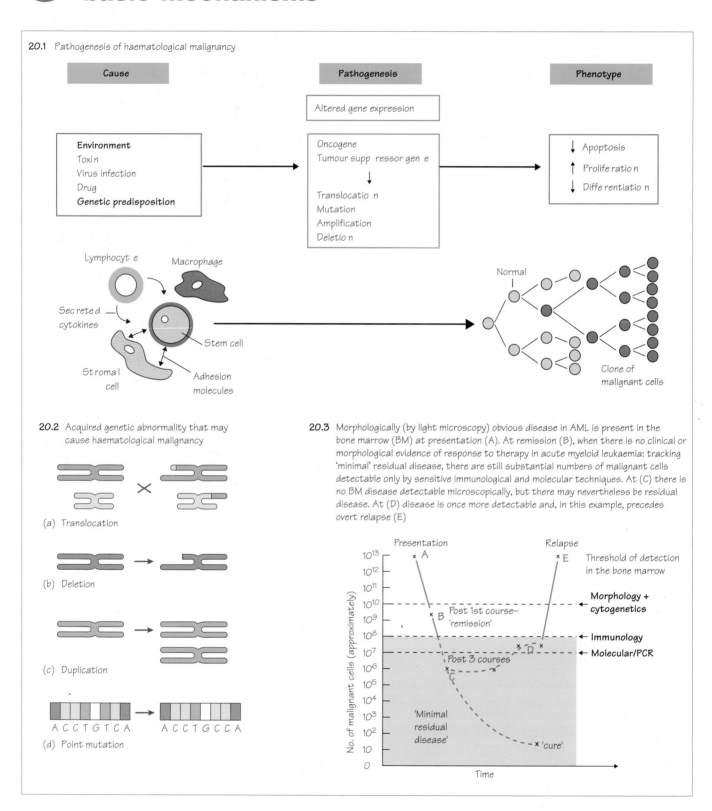

20.1 Pathogenesis of haematological malignancy

| Cause | Pathogenesis | Phenotype |

Altered gene expression

Environment
Toxin
Virus infection
Drug
Genetic predisposition

Oncogene
Tumour suppressor gene
↓
Translocation
Mutation
Amplification
Deletion

↓ Apoptosis
↑ Proliferation
↓ Differentiation

Lymphocyte
Macrophage
Secreted cytokines
Stem cell
Stromal cell
Adhesion molecules

Normal
Clone of malignant cells

20.2 Acquired genetic abnormality that may cause haematological malignancy

(a) Translocation

(b) Deletion

(c) Duplication

A C C T G T C A → A C C T G C C A

(d) Point mutation

20.3 Morphologically (by light microscopy) obvious disease in AML is present in the bone marrow (BM) at presentation (A). At remission (B), when there is no clinical or morphological evidence of response to therapy in acute myeloid leukaemia: tracking 'minimal' residual disease, there are still substantial numbers of malignant cells detectable only by sensitive immunological and molecular techniques. At (C) there is no BM disease detectable microscopically, but there may nevertheless be residual disease. At (D) disease is once more detectable and, in this example, precedes overt relapse (E).

Presentation — A
Relapse — E

Threshold of detection in the bone marrow

10^{13}
10^{12}
10^{11}
10^{10} — — — Morphology + cytogenetics
10^9 — B — Post 1st course—'remission'
10^8 — → Immunology
10^7 — D — → Molecular/PCR
10^6 — Post 3 courses
10^5 — C
10^4
10^3
10^2
10 — 'cure'
0

No. of malignant cells (approximately)

'Minimal residual disease'

Time

Haematology at a Glance, Fourth Edition. Atul B. Mehta and A. Victor Hoffbrand.

20.4 (a) Bone marrow biopsy form a patient with myeloma, showing characteristic plasma cells. The plasma cell nature of the cells is confirmed by demonstrating positive staining by immunocytochemistry with the CD 138 antigen 3b (b). The clonal nature of the cells is confirmed by demonstrating that the cells are positive for anti – kappa (c) but negative for anti lambda (d)

(a)

(b)

(c)

(d)

Neoplasia

Haematological malignancies (Table 20.1) are thought to arise from a single cell in the bone marrow, thymus or peripheral lymphoid system that has undergone one or more genetic change (somatic mutation) leading to malignant *transformation*. Successive mitotic divisions give rise to a clone of cells derived from the parent cell. Further mutations may give rise to subclones (clonal evolution). Transformed cells proliferate excessively and/or are resistant to apoptosis. They are often 'frozen' at a particular stage of differentiation. 'Acute' haematological malignancies are those that appear and progress over a short timescale (days or weeks) and the tumour cells are usually morphologically immature ('blasts'). They require immediate treatment. Chronic haematological malignancies appear and may remain stationary or progress over a longer timescale (months or years), and the tumour cells are often difficult to distinguish morphologically from normal cells; they may remain indolent and do not always require treatment.

Table 20.1 Classification of haematological malignancies (major types)

	Acute	Chronic
Lymphoid	Acute lymphoblastic leukaemia	Chronic lymphocytic leukaemia and variants
		Non-Hodgkin lymphoma (many different types)
		Hodgkin lymphoma
		Multiple myeloma and variants
Myeloid	Acute myeloid leukaemia	Chronic myeloid leukaemia
		Myelodysplasia
		Myeloproliferative disorders (polycythaemia vera, essential thrombocythaemia, primary myelofibrosis)

Causes of neoplasia

Neoplasia is caused by a complex interaction between genetic and environmental mechanisms (Fig. 20.1).

• Genetic predisposition. Certain inherited conditions predispose to haematological malignancy, e.g. Down syndrome, trisomy 21 and conditions associated with defective DNA repair, e.g. Fanconi anaemia, or immune suppression, e.g. ataxia telangiectasia. There are also single nucleotide polymorphisms present at birth of certain genes which predispose to haematological malignancies.

• Viral infection. Human T-cell leukaemia virus incorporates into T-lymphoid cell genome and underlies adult T-cell leukaemia lymphoma (see Chapter 33). Other viruses predispose to malignancy by immune suppression (e.g. HIV). Epidemiological evidence implicates Epstein–Barr virus (EBV) in Burkitt lymphoma and less strongly with Hodgkin lymphoma. EBV is also implicated in many post-transplant (usually of solid organs) lymphoproliferative diseases. *Helicobacter pylori* infection of the stomach predisposes to gastric lymphoma. Malaria predisposes to Burkitt lymphoma in tropical Africa.

• Ionizing radiation causes DNA mutation and increases the risk of haematological neoplasia.

• Toxins/chemicals, e.g. benzene and organochemicals, also alter DNA and may predispose to leukaemia and myelodysplasia (MDS).

• Drugs. Alkylating agents (e.g. melphalan, cylophosphamide) and other forms of chemotherapy predispose to MDS or acute myeloid leukaemia.

• In most cases of haematological malignancy, it remains unclear why any one individual develops it.

Mechanism of malignant transformation

Altered expression of two types of gene, oncogenes or tumour suppressive genes, underlies multistep pathogenesis of haematological malignancy.

Oncogenes

Oncogenes, whose protein products cause malignant transformation, are derived from normal cellular genes (proto-oncogenes). These code for proteins usually involved in one or other stage in cell signal transduction, gene transcription, the cell cycle, cell survival/apoptosis or differentiation. Often, the genes involved are tyrosine kinases that are involved in signal transduction in cells by phosphorylation of downstream proteins on tyrosine residues. Activation of proto-oncogenes to become oncogenes may occur by **amplification**, **point mutation** or **translocation** from one chromosomal location to another (Fig. 20.2).

Translocation is most frequent in haematological malignancies and may lead to a quantitative change in expression, (e.g. MYC translocation to the immunoglobulin heavy chain locus in lymphoid neoplasia, t(8;14) or of the *BCL-2* gene (which inhibits apoptosis) in follicular lymphoma t(14:18). Translocation may also lead to a qualitative change by joining all or part of the oncogene to another gene to form a fusion gene (e.g. *ABL-1* translocation from chromosome 9 to the breakpoint cluster region (BCR) on chromosome 22 to form the fusion gene *BCR-ABL1* in chronic myeloid leukaemia t(9;22) (see Chapter 24)).

Point mutation of JAK2, a signal transduction protein (see Fig. 26.1), is now known to underlie most cases of polycythaemia vera and about 50% of patients with other types of myeloproliferative disease (see Chapter 26).

Anti-oncogenes (tumour suppressor genes)

These are genes encoding proteins that have a critical role in suppressing cell growth. Chromosome deletion may obliterate tumour suppressor genes on one allele; deletion or mutation of the remaining allele may then allow uncontrolled cell growth.

Micro-RNAs

Micro-RNAs are synthesised from genes distributed throughout the genome. They affect transcription of other genes and may be deleted, e.g. in the 13q deletion in chronic lymphocytic leukaemia. Their deletion affects expression of other genes.

Evidence of clonality

A population of cells is considered clonal (derived from a single cell by mitotic division) if they have one or more of the following features.

• The identical acquired chromosome abnormality, e.g. Ph chromosome (Fig. 24.1) or point mutation within an individual gene.

• Clonal rearrangement of an immunoglobulin or T-cell receptor gene in lymphoid neoplasia (see Chapter 7).

• Restriction in a B-lymphoid neoplasm to expression of only λ or only κ light chains, but not both as in polyclonal B cells (Fig. 20.3). The cells may secrete a paraprotein (gammaglobulin made up of identical molecules).

Minimal residual disease

At the time of diagnosis of a haematological neoplasm, the patient will have approximately 10^{13}–10^{14} malignant cells. Even if treatment results in 1000-fold reduction of tumour cells, there remain 10^{10} cells, which may be below the microscopic level of detection. Using immunological or molecular techniques, minimal residual disease (MRD) may be detected in blood or marrow of patients who clinically, and by conventional light microscopy of blood and bone marrow, are in complete remission (Fig. 20.4).

The techniques to detect MRD include the following:

• Immunological (e.g. flow cytometry) if residual malignant cells carry a distinctively abnormal phenotype (pattern of antigen expression) (see Chapter 7).

• Chromosomal analysis and, more sensitively, fluorescence *in situ* hybridization (FISH) (see Chapter 7).

• Molecular using the polymerase chain reaction, e.g. for a particular B- or T-cell receptor gene rearrangement. This is the most sensitive (will detect one malignant cell in up to 10^5 normal cells).

21.1 Apheresis

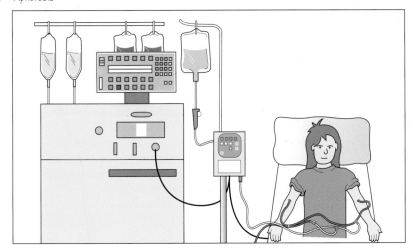

21.2 Acute leukaemia: Hickman line infection, which has rapidly evolved to septicaemia, and bloodborne skin lesions caused by coagulase-negative staphylococci

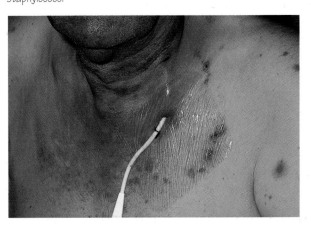

Haematology at a Glance, Fourth Edition. Atul B. Mehta and A. Victor Hoffbrand.
61

Chemotherapy

Chemotherapy is the use of pharmacological agents (Table 21.1) to treat malignant or other proliferative diseases. It may be given orally, by intravenous bolus, prolonged subcutaneous or intravenous injection/infusion or intrathecally. It may be a single agent or combination of chemotherapy-utilizing drugs with different, preferably synergistic, modes of action, with limited or no overlapping toxicity, and aimed at delaying emergence of drug resistance. Chemotherapy drugs are often given as a cycle of a few days' treatment every 3–6 weeks to allow normal cells, especially of the bone marrow and gastrointestinal tract, to recover from toxicity. Extravasation into tissues can cause severe local reactions. Intravenous chemotherapy is usually given through a central line or through a tunnelled intravenous catheter (e.g. Hickman's) or indwelling chamber (e.g. Port-a-Cath).

Table 21.1 Chemotherapy agents

DNA binding	
Anthracyclines	Other
Daunorubicin	Mitoxantrone
Hydroxydaunorubicin	Bleomycin
Idarubicin	
Alkylating agents	
Cyclophosphamide	Melphalan
Ifosfamide	Nitrosoureas (BCNU, CCNU)
Chlorambucil	Busulfan
Mitotic inhibitors	
Vincristine	
Vindesine	
Vinblastine	
Antimetabolites	
Methotrexate	Cytosine arabinoside
Mercaptopurine	Hydroxycarbamide
Azathioprine	
Inhibitors of DNA repair enzymes	
Epipodophyllotoxins e.g. etoposide	
Antipurines	
Fludarabine	
Deoxycoformycin	
2-Chlorodeoxydenosine	
Proteosome inhibitor	
Bortezomib	
Others	
Corticosteroids	
L-Asparaginase	
Biological agents: interferon, thalidomide, lenalidomide, pomalidomide	
Monoclonal antibodies	
Rituximab	Anti-CD20 (benign and malignant
Ofatumumade	B lymphoid disorders)
Alemtuzumab	Anti-CD52 (lymphoproliferative disorders)
Gemtuzumab	Anti-CD33 (AML)
Brentazumab	Anti-CD30 (Hodgkin's lymphoma)
Eculizumab	Anti-complement C5 (PNH)

AML, acute myeloid leukaemia; PNH, paroxysmal nocturnal haemoglobinuria

Mechanism of action

Chemotherapy drugs generally affect DNA synthesis or repair and promote cellular apoptosis. Cycle-specific agents prevent DNA synthesis and act on the S phase of the cell cycle (Table 21.1). Non-cycle-specific agents act at all phases of the cell cycle and include alkylating agents, which bind to DNA, and anthracyclines, which cause DNA strand breaks. Inhibition of the DNA repair enzyme, topoisomerase II, is an important component of the action of anthracyclines and etoposide.

Dose-dependent side effects of chemotherapy

Most chemotherapeutic agents are toxic to normal dividing cells (haemopoietic cells, gastrointestinal tract, hair, skin) as well as to malignant cells. Common side effects include the following:
- Bone marrow failure (anaemia, thrombocytopenia, neutropenia) with increased susceptibility to bleeding and infection, which may require therapy with antimicrobials, blood components and growth factors (granulocyte colony-stimulating factor (G-CSF), erythropoietin) and synthetic thrombomimetics.
- Nausea and vomiting requiring antiemetic therapy – metoclopramide, dexamethasone and 5-HT antagonists (e.g. ondansetron, granisetron).
- Mucositis (sore mouth and throat), abdominal pain and diarrhoea.
- Infertility – sperm storage considered *before* chemotherapy.
- Tumour lysis syndrome – prevented by good hydration, alkalinization of urine, allopurinol, rasburicase.
- Hyperuricaemia – prevented by allopurinol.
- Specific side effects of chemotherapy include neuropathy (vincristine), cardiomyopathy (anthracyclines), thrombosis (L-asparaginase, thalidomide), pulmonary fibrosis (busulfan, bleomycin) and haemorrhagic cystitis (cyclophosphamide).
- Secondary malignancy, e.g. myelodysplasia or acute leukaemia following alkylating agents or etoposide.
- Growth retardation in children.

Biological therapies

Growth factors in clinical use (see Chapter 1) include G-CSF, erythropoietin and synthetic analogues of thrombopoietin. The interferons are naturally occurring agents that have both antineoplastic and anti-infective properties. Monoclonal antibodies, e.g. rituximab (anti-CD20), alemtuzumab (anti-CD52) and gemtuzumab (anti-CD33), alone or bound to toxins or radioactive isotopes, may be used to kill specific cells or target drug therapy. Thalidomide and lenalidomide are used to treat myeloma, myelodysplasia and myelofibrosis.

Apheresis

Apheresis is a technique whereby whole blood is removed from the body and processed by centrifugation into its cellular components and plasma (Fig. 21.1). In plasma exchange, the plasma is removed and replaced by albumin (or fresh frozen plasma in thrombotic thrombocytopenia purpura; see Chapter 41). In *leucapheresis*, the white cells are removed. The process can also be used to perform a red cell exchange (e.g. in sickle cell disease), to remove platelets (platelet pheresis), to isolate lymphocytes for donation (donor lymphocyte infusion, e.g. for the treatment of relapse following a stem cell transplant) or to isolate haemopoietic stem cells (HSC) for donation (HSC transplantation).

Lumbar puncture

Cerebrospinal fluid is sampled from patients with haematological diseases for the following.

- Diagnosis – e.g. in case of infection, or infiltration by malignant cells.
- Treatment – e.g. malignancy (acute leukaemia, lymphoma) with intrathecal chemotherapy.

Lumbar puncture should only be undertaken in patients who have a platelet count >50 × 10⁹/L and after correction of coagulation abnormalities. Intrathecal chemotherapy should be prescribed and administered only by those who have appropriate training and experience.

Hickman line care

Indwelling lines that have been tunnelled under the skin and then into the subclavian vein (Fig. 21.2) allow easy venous access for blood sampling, administration of intravenous drugs, e.g. chemotherapy, antibiotics and feeding. All the ports must be kept patent when not in use by instillation of heparin. They should be sampled wearing gloves and using sterile technique. The first 5–10 mL of blood from each port must be discarded before samples are sent for testing. If the tube is blocked, the installation of urokinase or alteplase (tissue plasminogen activator) is used to dissolve the thrombus.

Infection

The main risk factors are as follow:
- Neutropenia (particularly if <0.5 × 10⁹/L) for bacterial and fungal infections.
- Organisms that are normal commensals may be pathogenic for immunocompromised patients.
- Defective cell-mediated or humoral immunity for viral, bacterial and atypical infections (e.g. tuberculosis).
- Others, such as indwelling catheters (intravenous, urethral), corticosteroid therapy and mucositis, also increase risk. Impaired splenic function or splenectomy reduces ability to make antibody, particularly to capsulated organisms, reduces clearance of intracellular organisms (e.g. parasitized red cells) and impairs defence against organisms and toxins in the portal circulation.

Organisms

- Bacterial – Gram-positive (coagulase-negative and -positive *Staphylococci*, *Streptococci*, *Enterococci*); Gram-negative (*Klebsiella*, *Pseudomonas*, *Escherichia coli*, *Proteus*); others, e.g. *Tuberculosis*, *atypical mycobacteria*;
- Fungal – *Candida*, *Aspergillus*;
- Viruses – *Cytomegalovirus*, *Herpes viruses*, *Adenoviruses*; and
- Protozoans – *Toxoplasma*, *Pneumocystis*, *Leishmania*, *Histoplasma*.

Prevention

- Good hygiene on the part of the patient and staff, regular hand cleaning and avoidance of contact with infected individuals.
- Barrier nursing in isolation is preferred. Staff wear gowns and gloves when in contact with severely neutropenic patients.
- Filtered air at positive pressure reduces risk from fungal spores.
- Food should ideally be cooked. Foods frequently contaminated with bacteria (soft cheeses, uncooked eggs and meat, salads, live yoghurt) are avoided and only peeled fruits are allowed.
- Oral non-absorbable antibiotics (e.g. neomycin, colistin) will reduce colonization of the gastrointestinal tract; oral systemic antibiotics (cip-

rofloxacin, co-trimoxazole) reduce the incidence of bacteraemia and oral antifungals (fluconazole amphotericin/itraconazole/posaconazole) and/or oral antiviral (aciclovir) prophylaxis are routinely given in some units for selected patients.

Diagnosis

- Fever is the cardinal sign of infection; tachycardia, tachypnoea, fall in blood pressure, cough, dysuria and altered mental state may also occur.
- Physical signs include reddened throat, inflamed intravenous catheter site, skin rash, chest signs, mouth signs and perineal inflammation. Pus is absent in neutropenic patients.
- Special tests to identify the responsible organism include microbial culture (sputum, urine, throat and perineal swab, blood cultures from peripheral blood and indwelling catheter, lumbar puncture – if neurological symptoms – skin swabs, faecal culture). Bronchoalveolar lavage may be necessary. Serological and molecular tests for specific organisms, e.g. *Candida*, *Aspergillus*, may be of value. Imaging tests may include chest X-ray, CT scan, especially of chest if fungal infection is suspected, and sinus X-rays.

Treatment

- Supportive care for renal failure/hypotension/respiratory failure.
- Empirical antibacterial therapy should be commenced in patients who are neutropenic (<0.5 × 10⁹/L) or otherwise severely immunocompromised and develop fever (temperature of 38°C or greater lasting for more than 2 h). Cultures should be taken and intravenous antibiotics should be commenced, with either a single, potent broad-spectrum agent (e.g. a fourth-generation cephalosporin or ureidopenicillin) or a combination of agents with activity against Gram-negative and Gram-positive (including coagulase-negative *Staphylococci*) organisms.
- Failure to respond should prompt treatment of atypical infections, e.g. fungi, viruses. Empirical antifungal treatment with liposomal amphotericin/voriconozole/caspofungin is required in high-risk patients, particularly after stem cell transplantation.

Radiotherapy

Ionizing radiation, usually derived from an external source, is used to treat disease by causing DNA damage in malignant cells. It is commonly used in the treatment of haematological malignancies (e.g. lymphoid leukaemias, lymphoma, myeloma) and as part of conditioning therapy for bone marrow transplant for malignant disease. Side effects include nausea, vomiting, alopecia, bone marrow failure, damage to normal tissues (e.g. skin burns), growth retardation and induction of second malignancies.

Counselling

Counselling is valuable for various groups of haematological patients.
- Patients and families with malignant disease need emotional support during treatment and/or bereavement. Practical help with housing, transport and welfare benefits should also be given. There should be good liaison with GPs, palliative and terminal care support teams in the community and hospices.

22.1 T-cell acute lymphoblastic leukaemia (T-ALL): bone marrow showing large numbers of lymphoblasts with a high nuclear/cytoplasmic ratio

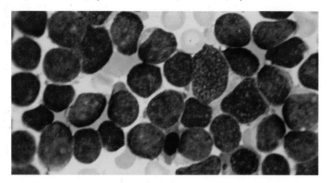

22.2 (a) Precursor B-cell ALL: bone marrow showing large blasts with characteristic vacuoles and blue cytoplasm

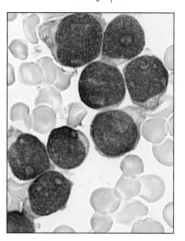

(b) Precursor B-ALL: cerebrospinal fluid cytocentrifuge specimen showing lymphoblasts

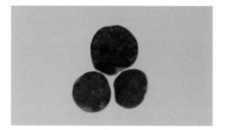

Haematology at a Glance, Fourth Edition. Atul B. Mehta and A. Victor Hoffbrand.

64 © 2014 John Wiley & Sons, Ltd. Published 2014 by John Wiley & Sons, Ltd. Companion Website: www.ataglanceseries.com/haematology

22.3 Acute myeloid leukaemia without maturation: bone marrow

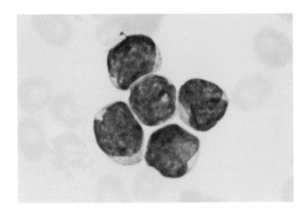

22.4 Acute myeloid leukaemia with maturation: bone marrow. Note Auer rod in myoblast

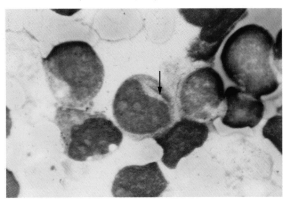

22.5 Acute promyelocytic leukaemia t(15;17): bone marrow. Note cell with multiple Auer rods (arrow)

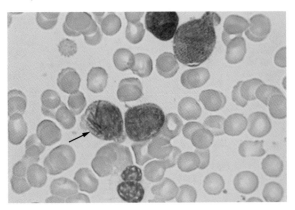

22.6 Acute monoblastic and monocytic leukaemia: bone marrow showing vacuolated monoblasts

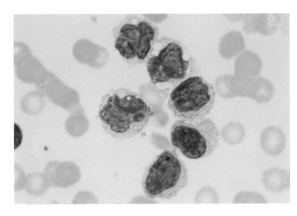

22.7 Acute erythroid leukaemia: bone marrow showing abnormal erythroid cells, erythroblasts and myeloblasts

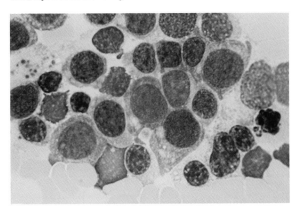

22.8 Acute megakaryoblastic leukaemia: bone marrow showing myeloblasts and megakaryoblasts, with platelets budding from the cytoplasm

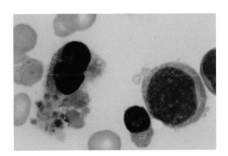

Acute leukaemia is a malignant disorder in which haemopoietic blast cells constitute >20% of bone marrow cells. The primitive cells usually also accumulate in the blood, infiltrate other tissues and cause bone marrow failure.

Classification

There are two main groups: acute lymphoblastic (ALL) and acute myeloid (myeloblastic) leukaemia (AML). Rare cases are undifferentiated or mixed. Subclassification of ALL or AML depends on morphological, immunological, cytogenetic and molecular criteria (Boxes 22.1 and 22.2; Table 22.1).

Aetiology and pathogenesis

The malignant cells typically show a chromosome translocation or other DNA mutation affecting oncogenes (see Chapter 20). AML may be primary or secondary; it may follow a previous myeloproliferative or myelodysplastic disease. In childhood B lineage (precursor B) ALL there is evidence from identical twin studies that the first event, a chromosomal translocation, may occur *in utero* and a subsequent second event (e.g. infection) precipitates the onset of ALL.

Incidence

There are approximately 1000 new cases (20–25 per million population) each of AML and ALL per year in the UK. ALL is the most common malignancy in childhood (peak age of 4 year) but also occurs in adults. AML occurs at all ages. It is rarer than ALL in childhood, being most common in the elderly.

Clinical features

- Short (<3 months) history of symptoms due to bone marrow failure (e.g. of anaemia, abnormal bruising/bleeding or infection). Disseminated intravascular coagulation (DIC) with bleeding is particularly common in promyelocytic AML t(15;17).
- Increased cellular catabolism may cause sweating, fever, weight loss and general malaise.

• Lymphadenopathy and hepatosplenomegaly are frequent, especially in ALL.
• Tissue infiltration, e.g. of meninges, testes (more common in ALL), skin, bones, gums with hypertrophy (AML with monocytic differentiation) may cause clinical symptoms or signs.

Laboratory features

• Anaemia, thrombocytopenia and often neutropenia.
• Leucocytosis caused by blast cells in the blood usually occurs. Some cases show severe neutropenia without circulating blasts.
• The bone marrow shows infiltration by blast cells (>20% and often 80–90% of marrow cells) (Fig. 22.1).
• Coagulation may be abnormal and DIC can occur, especially with acute promyelocytic leukaemia.
• Serum uric acid, lactate dehydrogenase may be raised.
• Morphological analysis (ALL, Fig. 22.2; AML, Fig. 22.3) usually reveals cytoplasmic granules or Auer rods (condensations of granules) in AML.
• Immunophenotype analysis involves the use of antibodies and fluorescence-activated cell sorting (FACS) (see Chapter 7) to identify cell antigens (many termed clusters of differentiation or CD, see Appendix) which correlate with lineage and maturity (Table 22.1). Other antigens, e.g. TdT, and cytoplasmic immunoglobulin, which help in diagnosis, may be also be detected. The pattern of antigen expression may also be detected by immunohistological analysis of bone marrow trephine biopsy specimens (see Chapter 7).

Table 22.2 Prognostic factors in acute lymphoblastic leukaemia

	Good	Bad
Sex	Female	Male
Age	2–9 years	Adult
White cell count	Low (<10 × 10^9/L)	High (>50 × 10^9/L)
Chromosomes	Hyperdiploid*	t(9;22), t(4;11)
Extramedullary disease	Absent	Present
Speed of remission	4 weeks	>4 weeks
Clearance of peripheral blood blasts	1 week	>1 week
Minimal residual disease in bone marrow	Negative at 1–3 months	Positive at 3–6 months or more

* Hyperdiploid = more than 48 chromosomes in the blast cells. Normal = 46.

• Cytogenetic analysis of dividing cells (see Chapter 7) or using the more sensitive fluorescence *in situ* hybridization (FISH) analysis of dividing or non dividing cells (see Chapter 7) gives diagnostic and prognostic information (Box 22.2; Table 22.2).
• Cases with normal cytogenetics may be subclassified after DNA analysis into whether or not they show mutations detected only by molecular techniques of genes, e.g. *FLT3*. These mutations also have prognostic significance (Box 22.2).

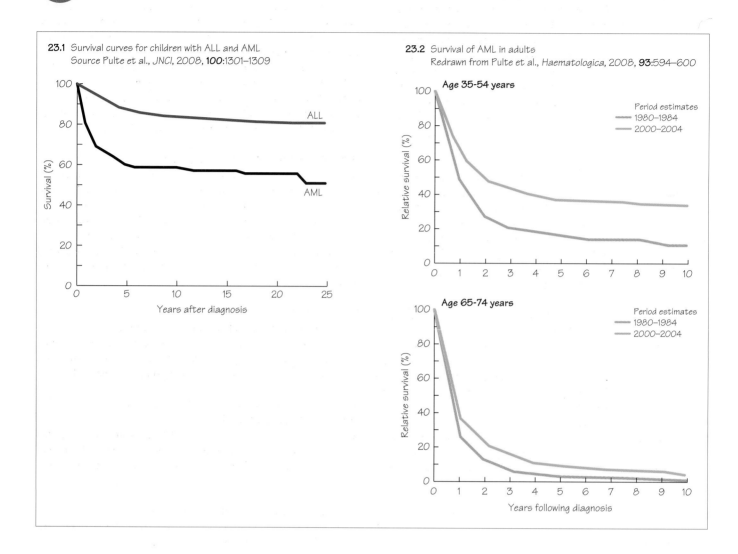

23.1 Survival curves for children with ALL and AML
Source Pulte et al., *JNCI*, 2008, **100**:1301–1309

23.2 Survival of AML in adults
Redrawn from Pulte et al., *Haematologica*, 2008, **93**:594–600

Age 35-54 years

Period estimates
1980–1984
2000–2004

Age 65-74 years

Period estimates
1980–1984
2000–2004

Haematology at a Glance, Fourth Edition. Atul B. Mehta and A. Victor Hoffbrand.

Treatment

The first phase of therapy (remission induction) is with high-dose intensive combination chemotherapy to reduce or eradicate leukaemic cells from the bone marrow and re-establish normal haemopoiesis. Further therapy is post-induction chemotherapy; this is initially intensive ('intensification' or 'consolidation' chemotherapy) and then, for acute lymphoblastic leukaemia (ALL) but not acute myeloid leukaemia (AML) less intensive (maintenance chemotherapy). Each course of intensive treatment typically requires 4–6 weeks in hospital. Complications of chemotherapy and supportive care are considered in Chapter 21; blood component therapy is considered in Chapter 49.

Acute myeloid leukaemia

Remission induction regimes usually comprise an anthracycline (e.g. daunorubicin), cytosine arabinoside (ara-C) and, in some protocols, etoposide. Fludarabine combined with high doses of ara-C and granulocyte colony-stimulating factor (G-CSF) (FLAG) may also be used for induction. All-*trans* retinoic acid (ATRA) is given with an anthracycline or arsenic trioxide in acute promyelocytic leukaemia (APML) to induce remission.

More than 80% of patients under the age of 60 years achieve remission, defined as a normal full blood count and <5% blasts in bone marrow, with one course and >85% with two courses. Older patients and those with preceding myelodysplasia or AML secondary to another disease (e.g. myeloproliferative disorder) have lower remission rates. Two or three further courses are usually given as post-induction therapy to younger (<60 years) patients, and other agents used include mitoxantrone, M-AMSA, idarubicin and high-dose ara-C. Tumour lysis syndrome may occur (see Chapter 21) and APML patients are at high risk of developing disseminated intravascular coagulation (DIC) (see Chapter 41). Anti-CD33 monoclonal antibody combined with a toxin (gemtuzumab) may be added in some AML protocols and recent evidence suggests that its inclusion increases overall survival. Some older patients may be considered medically unfit for intensive chemotherapy and may be treated with supportive care alone or with single agent, e.g. ara-C, hydroxycarbamide or low-dose gemtuzumab, chemotherapy.

Acute lymphoblastic leukaemia

Remission induction regimens comprise vincristine, dexamethasone and L-asparaginase, often with daunorubicin or cyclophosphamide.

Post-remission therapy is with two or three 'intensification' blocks with additional drugs. Patients then receive maintenance chemotherapy for a further 2–3 years with daily mercaptopurine, weekly methotrexate and monthly vincristine and dexamethasone. Treatment protocols may be modified according to whether minimal residual disease can be detected at various time points in therapy.

Central nervous system involvement is common in ALL in children and adults, and normal practice is to give multiple intrathecal injections of methotrexate to prevent this complication and courses of high-dose systemic chemotherapy with methotrexate or ara-C, or cranial radiotherapy to treat this complication if it occurs.

Stem cell transplantation (see Chapter 38)

Allogeneic stem cell transplantation (SCT) is recommended for selected (according to risk of relapse) adult patients (<60 years) in first remission of AML and for adults with ALL (>20 years and <50 years) who have a poor prognosis and histocompatible sibling. Transplants using matched unrelated volunteer donors are being increasingly performed. However, good prognosis AML (see Table 22.1) and good prognosis ALL (see Table 22.2) cases are not given SCT in first remission.

Prognosis

Childhood acute lymphoblastic leukaemia

Overall, 80% of children with ALL are cured, the best responses being in girls, aged 2–12 years with low presenting white cell count (<10 × 10^9/L) and favourable cytogenetics (Fig 23.1; see Table 22.2).

Acute myeloid leukaemia and adult acute lymphoblastic leukaemia

Approximately 30–50% of patients aged 15–55 years are cured. This varies according to age and prognostic features. Results are improving in the 55–64 year group, but over 75 years less than 5% are cured (Fig. 23.2).

Long-term complications of treatment

Increasing cure rates mean that long-term complications are relevant for all children and most adults (see Chapter 21).

24 Chronic myeloid leukaemia (*BCR-ABL1* positive)

24.1 The Philadelphia chromosome is an abnormal chromosome 22 caused by translocation of part of its long arm (q) to chromosome 9, and reciprocal translocation of part of chromosome 9, including the ABL1 oncogene, to a breakpoint cluster region (BCR) of chromosome 22. A fusion gene results on the derived chromosome 22, which leads to the synthesis of an abnormal protein with tyrosine protein kinase activity that is much greater than that of the normal ABL1 protein

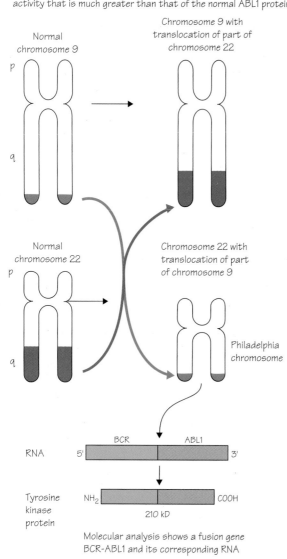

Normal chromosome 9

Chromosome 9 with translocation of part of chromosome 22

p

q

Normal chromosome 22

Chromosome 22 with translocation of part of chromosome 9

p

q

Philadelphia chromosome

RNA

BCR   ABL1

5'   3'

Tyrosine kinase protein

NH₂   COOH

210 kD

Molecular analysis shows a fusion gene BCR-ABL1 and its corresponding RNA

24.2 Chronic myeloid leukaemia (chronic phase): peripheral blood film, showing immature granulocytes (myelocytes, metamyelocytes) in the peripheral blood

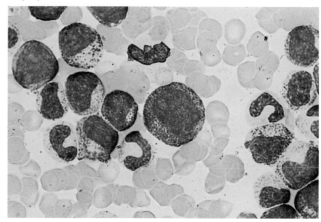

24.3 Chronic myeloid leukaemia: levels of detection of disease by morphology, cytogenetics and reverse transcriptase (RQ)-PCR following tyrosine kinase inhibitor therapy

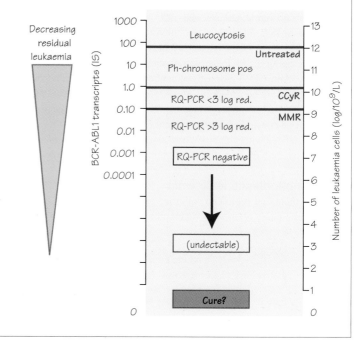

Decreasing residual leukaemia

BCR-ABL1 transcripts (IS)

1000
100
10
1.0
0.10
0.01
0.001
0.0001

Number of leukaemia cells (log/10⁹/L)

13
12
11
10
9
8
7
6
5
4
3
2
1

Leucocytosis

Untreated

Ph-chromosome pos

RQ-PCR <3 log red.   CCyR

RQ-PCR >3 log red.   MMR

RQ-PCR negative

(undectable)

Cure?

Haematology at a Glance, Fourth Edition. Atul B. Mehta and A. Victor Hoffbrand.

This is a clonal myeloproliferative disorder characterized by an increase in neutrophils and their precursors in the peripheral blood with increased cellularity of the marrow as a result of an excess of granulocyte precursors. The leukaemic cells of patients have a reciprocal translocation between the long arms of chromosomes 9 and 22, t(9;22). The derived chromosome 22 is termed the Philadelphia (Ph) chromosome (Fig. 24.1). Molecular analysis shows a fusion gene BCR-ABL1 and its corresponding RNA. The disease may transform from a relatively stable chronic phase to an acute leukaemia phase (blast transformation).

Aetiology and pathophysiology

Aetiology is unknown. Exposure to ionizing radiation is a risk factor. The ABL1 gene is translocated from chromosome 9 into the breakpoint cluster region (BCR) on chromosome 22 to form the BCR-ABL1 fusion gene (Fig. 24.1). This fusion gene encodes a 210-kDa protein with greatly increased tyrosine kinase activity compared to the normal ABL1 product. The disease is of stem cell origin as the Ph chromosome is present in erythroid, granulocytic, megakaryocytic and T-lymphoid precursors. Rare cases show variant translocations or are Ph-negative but show the BCR-ABL1 fusion gene. The Ph chromosome abnormality may also occur in acute lymphoblastic leukaemia (ALL; see Chapter 22).

Clinical features

• The disease occurs at all ages (peak age of 25–45 years, male : female ratio equal, incidence of 5–10 cases per million population).
• Patients usually present in the chronic phase.
• Presenting symptoms include weight loss, night sweats, itching, left hypochondrial pain, gout.
• Priapism, visual disturbance and headaches caused by hyperviscosity (WBC $>250 \times 10^9$/L) are less frequent.
• Splenomegaly, often massive, occurs in over 90% of cases.
• Some cases are discovered on a routine blood test.

Laboratory findings

• Raised white cell count (often 50×10^9/L or more), mainly neutrophils and myelocytes (Fig. 24.2).
• Basophils may be prominent.
• Platelet count may be raised, normal or low and anaemia may be present.
• Raised serum uric acid.
• Bone marrow is hypercellular with a raised myeloid : erythroid ratio (see Chapter 1).
• Cytogenetic analysis of bone marrow cells shows the Ph chromosome in >95% of metaphases. The BCR-ABL1 fusion gene is (by definition) detectable in 100% of cases by fluororescence in situ hydridization (FISH) and its RNA product by polymerase chain reaction (PCR; see Chapter 7).

Course and progress

Patients are typically well during the chronic phase. Main cause of death is transformation into acute leukaemia (80% AML, 20% ALL, with a proportion showing a mixed blast cell population), which may occur at any stage, even at presentation. The introduction of specific tyrosine kinase inhibitor drugs has transformed the outlook and overall survival rates are over 90% at 7 years after diagnosis. Staging based on age, spleen size, blood blast cell and platelet count can be used to predict outcome. There may be an accelerated phase of variable duration in which anaemia, thrombocytopenia, splenic enlargement and marrow fibrosis occur. Transformation is usually accompanied by additional morphological and chromosome abnormalities.

Treatment

Chronic phase

Imatinib (Glivec)

• This is a specific inhibitor of the tyrosine kinase encoded by BCR-ABL1. Treatment improves the blood count and causes the marrow to become Ph-negative in a high proportion of cases (Fig. 24.3); the patients with the best responses become negative for the BCR-ABL1 fusion gene when tested by PCR and >95% will still be alive 10 years after diagnosis. The duration of the chronic phase is prolonged in nearly all patients and rate of acute transformation is greatly reduced. Side effects include nausea, skin rashes and muscle pains. Imatinib in combination with other drugs is also valuable in therapy of Ph-positive ALL and blast transformation of chronic myeloid leukaemia (CML).
• Other tyrosine kinase inhibitors include nilotinib and dasatinib. They may be more active than imatinib in patients with acute transformation. They also have activity in patients with CML who become resistant to imatinib. Trials suggest they may also be more effective than imatinib as initial therapy.
• Imatinib and the newer drugs have made a major impact on the prognosis for patients with CML. If imatinib therapy is discontinued in patients in whom BCR-ABL1 RNA is no longer detectable in blood, about 50% will remain negative and in 50% will become positive again for BCR-ABL1.
• Hydroxycarbamide (hydroxyurea) will control the raised white cell count and may be used initially before starting imatinib.
• α-Interferon (IFN) may also control the white cell count and may delay onset of acute transformation, prolonging overall survival by 1–2 years. The best responders to IFN become Ph-negative, but usually remain BCR-ABL1-positive.
• Allopurinol to prevent hyperuricaemia.
• Allogeneic stem cell transplantation (SCT) is reserved for the minority of patients who do not respond to tyrosine kinase inhibitors or are already in accelerated or acute phase at presentation. Human leucocyte antigen (HLA) matched unrelated donor SCT is less successful in curing the disease because of higher morbidity and mortality. Transfusion of donor lymphocytes may be valuable in eliminating BCR-ABL1-positive cells in case of relapse post-SCT.

Acute phase

This is now much rarer with the widespread use of tyrosine kinase inhibitors.

Therapy as for acute leukaemia, AML or ALL with addition of a tyrosine kinase inhibitor e.g. dasatinib or nilotinib may be given; SCT may also be tried but the prognosis is poor.

Rare variants of CML include chronic neutrophilic eosinophilic and basophilic leukaemias. These are BCR-ABL1-negative and generally do not respond to imatinib.

25 Myelodysplasia (myelodysplastic syndromes)

25.1 Myelodysplasia: peripheral blood film showing hypogranular neutrophils with bilobed nuclei (pseudo-Pelger cells)

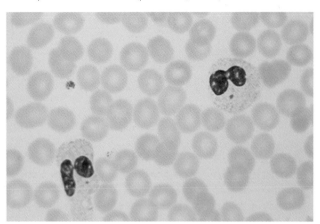

25.2 Myelodysplasia: bone marrow aspirate showing a granular blast with blue cytoplasm (arrow) and hypogranular maturing myeloid cells

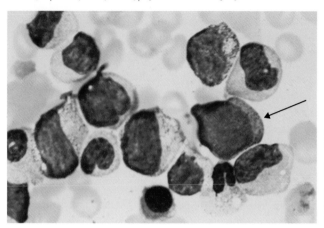

25.3 Myelodysplasia: bone marrow aspirate showing mononuclear and binuclear micromegakaryocytes

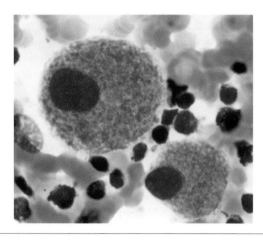

25.4 Iron (Perls') stain of bone marrow aspirate showing iron granules in a perinuclear distribution (ringed sideroblasts) from a patients with myelodysplasia

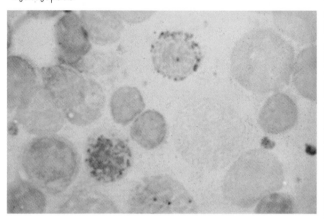

Haematology at a Glance, Fourth Edition. Atul B. Mehta and A. Victor Hoffbrand.

72 © 2014 John Wiley & Sons, Ltd. Published 2014 by John Wiley & Sons, Ltd. Companion Website: www.ataglanceseries.com/haematology

Myelodysplasia (MDS) is a clonal haemopoietic stem cell disorder characterized by peripheral blood cytopenias most frequently affecting more than one lineage usually in association with a hypercellular marrow indicating ineffective haemopoiesis.

Aetiology and pathogenesis

MDS may be primary (*de novo*) or a consequence of previous chemotherapy/radiotherapy (secondary). Various chromosome abnormalities occur, e.g. complete or partial deletions of chromosomes 5 or 7. Point mutations detected by molecular techniques are frequent, e.g. in *RAS* or other oncogenes. Mutation of genes involved in RNA splicing occur in 45–85% of cases of MDS. The disease is divided into six subgroups or myelodysplastic syndromes largely depending on how many bone marrow lineages are involved, whether or not 'ring sideroblasts' are present in the bone marrow and the proportion of myeloblasts in the marrow (Figure 25.1d; Box 25.1). It may transform to acute myeloid leukaemia (AML) (>20% blasts in the marrow).

Clinical features

• Most frequent in the elderly, but young adults or even children may be affected.
• Bone marrow failure (see Chapter 36) with anaemia and/or leucopenia and/or thrombocytopenia.
• The 5q-syndrome is a subgroup, occurring particularly in elderly females with an elevated platelet count, macrocytosis and good prognosis.

Laboratory findings

• Anaemia is usually macrocytic.
• Neutropenia is frequent and neutrophils may be hypogranular with reduced lobulation of the nucleus (pseudo-Pelger forms; Fig. 25.1a).
• Bone marrow is usually hypercellular but may be hypocellular and/or fibrotic.
• Characteristic morphological changes are usually seen in all three (erythroid, granulocyte and megakaryocyte) lineages (Fig. 25.1a–c).
• Ring sideroblasts (erythroid precursors with iron granules forming a ring around the nucleus) form >15% of erythroblasts in some types (Box 25.1).

Differential diagnosis

This is very broad, particularly when only one lineage is involved in an elderly person. Thus, other causes of anaemia (e.g. B$_{12}$ or folate deficiency, chronic inflammation, myeloma) must be excluded. Thrombocytopenia or leucopenia may be caused by drugs, immune destruction or hypersplenism. The hallmark of MDS is involvement of more than one – typically all three – lineage(s). Nevertheless, distinction between MDS, myelofibrosis and aplastic anaemia may be difficult in patients with pancytopenia. The finding of a cytogenetic abnormality greatly strengthens what may otherwise be a subjective morphological diagnosis of MDS.

Course and prognosis

This depends on the type of MDS (Box 25.1). The degree of cytopenia influences the incidence of complications and treatment, while the percentage of blast cells is predictive of the risk of developing acute leukaemia. The presence of complex cytogenetic changes is also associated with a poor prognosis. Scoring systems have been devised whereby the degree of cytopenia, proportion of blasts and nature of

> ### Box 25.1 Classification of the myelodysplastic and myelodysplastic/myeloproliferative syndromes
>
> **Myelodysplastic syndromes**
> Refractory cytopenias with unilineage dysplasia
>   Refractory anaemia
>   Refractory neutropenia
>   Refractory thrombocytopenia
> Refractory anaemia with ring sideroblasts
> Refractory cytopenia with multilineage dysplasia
> Refractory anaemia with excess marrow blasts: type I (5–9%), type II (10–19%)
> Myelodysplastic syndromes associated with isolated del (5q)
>
> **Myelodysplastic/myeloproliferative neoplasms**
> Chronic myelomonocytic leukaemia
> Atypical chronic myeloid leukaemia, *BCR-ABL1*-negative
> Juvenile myelomonocytic leukaemia

cytogenetic changes are used to estimate prognosis. These scoring systems are helpful in planning treatment as they help in making complex decisions whereby the risks of treatment must be balanced against the risk of disease progression. Death may be caused by infection, haemorrhage, iron overload from multiple transfusions or from transformation into AML.

Treatment

• Support care with red cell or platelet transfusions and antimicrobials may be required.
• Erythropoietin produces a rise in haemoglobin in about 5–15% of patients with refractory anaemia. Granulocyte colony-stimulating factor (G-CSF) has been used to increase neutrophil production temporarily if an infection is present.
• Iron chelation therapy may be needed for multiply transfused iron loaded patients with an otherwise good prognosis.
• Chemotherapy with low-dose ara-C, etoposide, hydroxycarbamide or 6-mercaptopurine is used to control excess blast proliferation in patients unsuitable for high-dose chemotherapy. Newer agents include azacitidine and dacarbazine. The thalidomide derivative lenalidomide is particularly active in patients with the 5q abnormality.
• Younger patients with refractory anaemia with excess blasts (RAEB) may be treated as for AML. Complete remissions are less frequent than in *de novo* AML.
• Allogeneic stem cell transplantation (sibling or matched unrelated donor) may cure younger patients. Reduced intensity transplants are performed in selected patients up to the age of 70 years.

Myelodysplastic/myeloproliferative diseases

These have many of the laboratory findings of MDS with a hypercellular marrow and dysplastic features in the different cell lineages. In chronic myelomonocytic leukaemia, there are >1.0 × 10^9/L monocytes in the peripheral blood, the spleen may be enlarged and marrow blasts are up to 10%. Juvenile myelomonocyte leukaemia is associated with lymphadenopathy and eczematous rash.

26.1

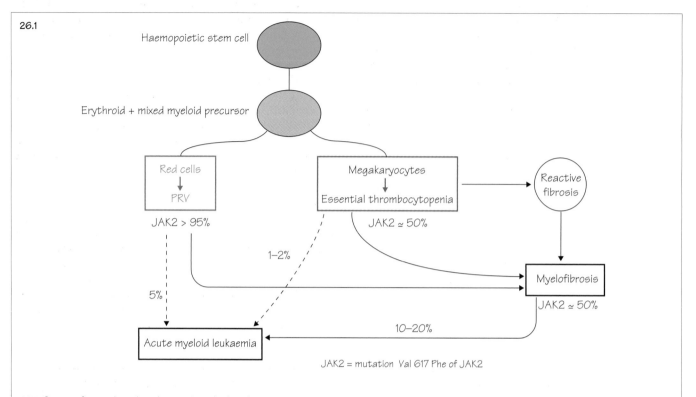

Haemopoietic stem cell

Erythroid + mixed myeloid precursor

Red cells
↓
PRV

JAK2 > 95%

Megakaryocytes
↓
Essential thrombocytopenia

JAK2 ≈ 50%

Reactive fibrosis

Myelofibrosis

JAK2 ≈ 50%

1–2%

5%

10–20%

Acute myeloid leukaemia

JAK2 = mutation Val 617 Phe of JAK2

26.2 Causes of secondary thrombocytosis and polycythaemia

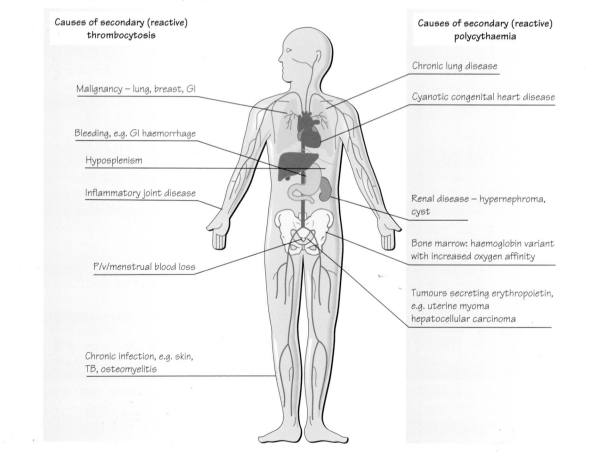

Causes of secondary (reactive) thrombocytosis

Malignancy – lung, breast, GI

Bleeding, e.g. GI haemorrhage

Hyposplenism

Inflammatory joint disease

P/v/menstrual blood loss

Chronic infection, e.g. skin, TB, osteomyelitis

Causes of secondary (reactive) polycythaemia

Chronic lung disease

Cyanotic congenital heart disease

Renal disease – hypernephroma, cyst

Bone marrow: haemoglobin variant with increased oxygen affinity

Tumours secreting erythropoietin, e.g. uterine myoma hepatocellular carcinoma

Haematology at a Glance, Fourth Edition. Atul B. Mehta and A. Victor Hoffbrand.

Myeloproliferative disorders (MPD) are chronic diseases caused by clonal proliferation of bone marrow stem cells usually leading to excess production of one or more haemopoietic lineage. The clinical syndromes include polycythaemia rubra vera (PRV) (red cells), essential thrombocythaemia (ET) (platelets) and primary myelofibrosis in which there is a reactive fibrosis of the marrow and extramedullary haemopoiesis in the liver and spleen. Intermediate forms may occur and the diseases may all transform into acute myeloid leukaemia. A mutation (Val617Phe) of the Janus kinase 2 (*JAK2*) is present in nearly 100% of cases of PRV and about 50% of cases of ET or primary myelofibrosis (Fig. 26.1). It is usually heterozygous, but homozygous in 5–10% of positive cases, and these tend to be clinically more severe. The mutation causes autonomous activation of signal transduction from the growth factor receptor for erythropoietin. This leads to uncontrolled cell proliferation. Chronic myeloid leukaemia was formerly classified as an MPD but is now known to be due to a different mutation (*BCR-ABL1*; see Chapter 24).

Differential diagnosis

Increased levels of red cells, white cells and platelets can occur in a range of physiological and reactive conditions. Reactive causes of increased levels of white cells are considered in Chapter 18; secondary or reactive causes of increased levels of red cells, platelets and of increased bone marrow fibrosis are listed in Boxes 26.1–26.3 and shown in Fig 26.2. Careful clinical assessment is required to distinguish these reactive (secondary) conditions from primary MPD in which there is an intrinsic disorder within the marrow stem cells. The general underlying mechanism for the secondary or reactive disorders is that an external stimulus leads to increased elaboration of erythropoietin and/or thrombopoietin (see Chapter 1). This leads to increased production of red cells and/or platelets by the bone marrow. This response may be physiological and appropriate (e.g. an increased haemoglobin level in response to tissue hypoxia, or an increased platelet count in response to haemorrhage) or it may be pathological (e.g. increased red cell and/or platelet counts in response to ectopic production of growth factors by tumours). The presence of a mutation within the *JAK2* locus or of a clonal cytogenetic abnormality confirms that the patient has a primary MPD.

Polycythaemia

Polycythaemia (erythrocytosis) is defined as an increase in haemoglobin concentration above normal (see Normal values). True polycythaemia exists when the red cell mass is increased above normal. Spurious (pseudo or stress) polycythaemia exists when an elevated haemoglobin concentration is caused by a reduction in plasma volume (see Chapter 27).

Thrombocytosis

Thrombocytosis is defined as an elevation of the blood platelet count above the normal range. Patients with thrombocytosis are at an increased risk of thrombosis but this is usually less when the underlying cause is reactive rather than an MPD. Treatment of secondary or reactive polycythaemia, thrombocytosis and increased marrow fibrosis is usually directed at the underlying cause. Patients with reactive thrombocytosis may also require treatment with antiplatelet agents, e.g. aspirin, to reduce the risk of thrombosis.

Box 26.1 Causes of polycythaemia

True polycythaemia
Primary
PRV

Congenital (rare)
Haemoglobin variant with increased oxygen affinity
Mutation in a renal oxygen sensing protein

Secondary
Erythropoietin appropriately increased
   High altitude
   Cyanotic congenital heart disease
   Chronic lung disease
   Haemoglobin variant with increased oxygen affinity
Erythropoietin inappropriately increased
   Renal disease: hypernephroma, renal cyst, hydronephrosis
   Uterine myoma
Other tumours, e.g. hepatocellular carcinoma, bronchial carcinoma

Relative polycythaemia
Pseudo ('stress') polycythaemia
Dehydration
Diuretic therapy

PRV, polycythaemia rubra vera

Box 26.2 Causes of an elevated platelet count

Primary
Essential thrombocythaemia
As part of another myeloproliferative disorder, e.g. PRV, CML, primary myelofibrosis

Reactive
Iron deficiency
Haemorrhage
Severe haemolysis
Trauma, postoperatively
Infection, inflammation
Malignancy
Hyposplenism

CML, chronic myeloid leukaemia; PRV, polycythaemia rubra vera

---

Box 26.3 Causes of marrow fibrosis

Primary

Secondary
Metastatic cancer
Acute leukaemia, especially megakaryocytic
Myelodysplasia
Hairy cell leukaemia
Connective tissue disease, e.g. systemic lupus erythematosus
Other, e.g. tuberculosis

Myeloproliferative disorders II: polycythaemia rubra vera

27.1 Polycythaemia rubra vera: patient with plethora

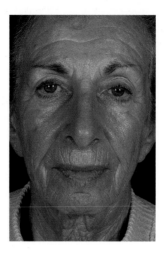

27.2 Polycythaemia rubra vera: clinical features

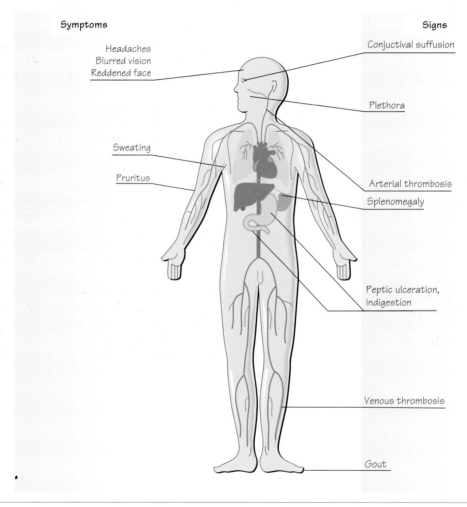

Symptoms

Headaches
Blurred vision
Reddened face

Sweating

Pruritus

Signs

Conjuctival suffusion

Plethora

Arterial thrombosis

Splenomegaly

Peptic ulceration, indigestion

Venous thrombosis

Gout

Haematology at a Glance, Fourth Edition. Atul B. Mehta and A. Victor Hoffbrand.

76 © 2014 John Wiley & Sons, Ltd. Published 2014 by John Wiley & Sons, Ltd. Companion Website: www.ataglanceseries.com/haematology

Polycythaemia rubra vera

Aetiology and pathophysiology

Polycythaemia rubra vera (PRV) is a primary neoplastic disorder in which bone marrow erythropoiesis is increased, usually accompanied by increased thrombopoiesis and granulopoiesis. Serum erythropoietin (EPO) levels are low. The *JAK2* gene product is a tyrosine kinase that has a key role in signal transduction (see Chapter 1). Mutation of *JAK2* is present in >95% of cases of PRV (and also in about 50% of cases with essential thrombocythaemia and primary myelofibrosis) (see Chapter 26). The mutation has the effect of amplifying the growth-promoting action of EPO. It is not clear why the same mutation underlies three different, although clearly related, diseases. The mutation is usually heterozygous, but in a minority it is homozygous and has a more profound effect.

Clinical features (Fig. 27.2)

- PRV occurs equally in males and females, typically over 55 years of age.
- Raised red cell mass (RCM) and blood volume causes a ruddy complexion (Fig. 27.1) and conjunctival suffusion; hyperviscosity may lead to headaches and visual disturbance.
- Thrombosis (e.g. deep vein thrombosis, Budd–Chiari syndrome, stroke) is also caused by hyperviscosity and increased platelets.
- Excess histamine secretion from basophils leads to increased gastric acid and peptic ulcer is frequent.
- Pruritus, typically after a hot bath.
- Haemorrhage, especially gastrointestinal, may occur.
- Enlarged spleen is found in 75% of patients and, if present, distinguishes PRV from other causes of polycythaemia (Fig. 26.2).
- Gout may occur due to increased cell turnover with uric acid production.

Laboratory features

- Raised haemoglobin concentration, haematocrit and red cell count.
- Seventy five per cent of patients have raised white cells (neutrophil leucocytosis) and/or platelets.
- *JAK2* mutation Val617Phe in >95% of patients; rare cases show other mutations in *JAK2*.
- Serum uric acid is usually raised.
- Serum lactic dehydrogenase is normal or slightly raised.
- Serum EPO is low.
- Bone marrow is hypercellular with prominent megakaryocytes, iron stores are depleted because of excessive iron incorporation into red cells and the trephine biopsy may show mildly increased reticulin.
- Abdominal ultrasound excludes renal disease and assesses spleen size.
- Culture of peripheral blood cells shows spontaneous formation of erythroid colonies in the absence of exogenous EPO.

Differential diagnosis

The *JAK2* mutation is absent in all other forms of polycythaemia. Secondary or reactive polycythaemia may occur in conditions where arterial oxygen saturation is reduced, leading to a physiological rise in serum EPO, or when EPO levels are inappropriately raised (e.g. caused by secretion of EPO by a renal neoplasm or other turmour) (see Fig. 26.2). Serum EPO measurement is indicated.

Treatment

- Thrombosis is the main cause of morbidity and mortality and its incidence can be reduced by maintaining the PCV around 0.45 or below and platelets below 600×10^9/L. Aspirin (75 mg/day) is used to inhibit platelet function.
- Multiple venesections are used initially to lower the PCV and in some cases for long-term treatment.
- Chemotherapy (e.g. oral hydroxycarbamide) is also usually required.
- Specific *JAK2*-inhibiting drugs are in clinical trial.
- A proton pump inhibitor is used for patients with indigestion or history of gastrointestinal bleeding.
- Allopurinol is used to prevent hyperuricaemia.

Prognosis

Median survival is about 16 years. Up to 30% of patients develop myelofibrosis (see Chapter 28). Acute myeloid leukaemia occurs in up to 5% of patients, not increased by hydroxycarbamide.

Spurious (pseudo) polycythaemia

The common form (at least 10 times more common than PRV) occurs particularly in young male adults, especially smokers, and may be associated with hypertension (Gaisböck's syndrome). The white cell and platelet counts are normal, as is the bone marrow and RCM. If the packed cell volume is over 0.50, it is treated by venesections to reduce the risk of cardiovascular complications; patients should reduce weight, stop smoking, moderate alcohol intake and avoid diuretics. Pseudopolycythaemia also may occur when plasma volume is reduced by dehydration, vomiting or diuretic therapy. Chest X-ray and arterial blood gas analysis to exclude lung disease are occasionally required.

Tests for congenital polycythaemia

1 Haemoglobin oxygen dissociation curve to identify a variant haemoglobin with increased oxygen affinity.
2 Mutation analysis of genes of proteins (HIF, VHL) concerned with oxygen sensing and erythropoietin production in the kidney.

28 Myeloproliferative disorders III: essential thrombocythaemia, primary myelofibrosis and systemic mastocytosis

28.1 Essential thrombocythaemia: peripheral blood film showing increased platelets with giant forms

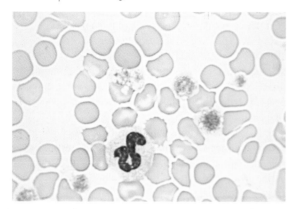

28.2 Primary myelofibrosis: peripheral blood film showing aniso/poikilocytosis, teardrop forms and giant platelets

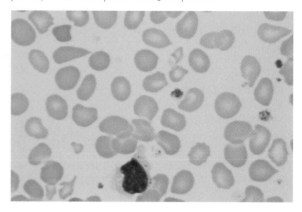

28.3 Primary myelofibrosis: bone marrow biopsy showing increased cellularity and large numbers of megakaryocytes

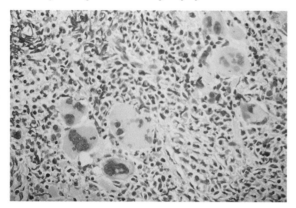

28.4 Primary myelofibrosis: bone marrow biopsy (reticulin stain) showing increased reticulin

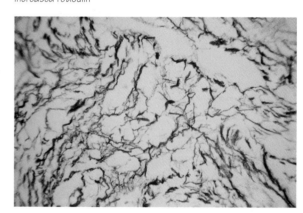

Essential thrombocythaemia

Essential thrombocythaemia (ET) is defined as persistent elevation of the peripheral blood platelet count (thrombocytosis) as a result of increased marrow platelet production in the absence of a systemic cause for thrombocytosis (see Box 26.2).

Aetiology and pathophysiology

It is similar to polycythaemia rubra vera (PRV), and distinction between the two conditions is not exact. ET occurs more frequently in younger adults than PRV. *JAK2* is mutated in 50% of cases.

Clinical features

- Thrombosis, both arterial (peripheral vessels with gangrene of toes, cerebral, coronary and mesenteric arteries) and venous (e.g. Budd–Chiari syndrome, deep vein thrombosis, superficial thrombophlebitis).
- Headaches, visual disturbance.
- At least 30% of patients are asymptomatic and detected as an incidental finding.
- Excessive haemorrhage may occur spontaneously or after trauma or surgery.
- Pruritus and sweating are uncommon.

Haematology at a Glance, Fourth Edition. Atul B. Mehta and A. Victor Hoffbrand.

• Splenomegaly in about 30% of patients; in others, the spleen is atrophied because of infarction.

Laboratory features
• Platelet count is persistently raised and often $>1000 \times 10^9$/L, raised red cell and/or white cell count is present in about 30%.
• Blood film shows platelet anisocytosis with circulating megakaryocyte fragments (Fig. 28.1). Autoinfarction of the spleen may cause changes in red cells (target cells, Howell–Jolly bodies).
• The *JAK2* mutation is present in about 50% of cases. In a few, this is homozygous and these tend to be more severe.
• Serum uric acid is often raised, serum lactic dehydrogenase is normal unless marrow fibrosis is present.
• Bone marrow is hypercellular with increased numbers of megakaryocytes, often in aggregates.

Treatment
• Younger patients (<40 years) with a platelet count $<1500 \times 10^9$/L, and no other risk factors for arterial or venous thrombosis may be treated with 75 mg/day aspirin alone. For patients aged 40–60 years, trials of aspirin alone against aspirin and hydroxycarbamide are in progress.
• Chemotherapy: hydroxycarbamide is used to reduce the platelet count in patients over 60 years.
• α-Interferon may be used in younger subjects but needs injections and has side effects (flu-like symptoms).
• Anagrelide is also effective but may cause cardiovascular or gastrointestinal side effects.
• Aspirin (75 mg/day), except in those with haemorrhage.
• *JAK2* inhibitors are in clinical trial.

Prognosis
Median survival is more than 20 years; thrombosis and haemorrhage are the main causes of morbidity and mortality. Transformation to acute myeloid leukaemia occurs in 1–5% of patients and to myelofibrosis in a higher proportion.

Primary myelofibrosis
Myelofibrosis (myelosclerosis, agnogenic myeloid metaplasia) is characterized by splenomegaly, extramedullary haemopoiesis, a leucoerythroblastic blood picture and replacement of bone marrow by collagen fibrosis. It must be distinguished from secondary causes of marrow fibrosis (see Box 26.3).

Aetiology and pathophysiology
Primary defect is within the haemopoietic stem cell; fibrosis results from a reactive non-neoplastic proliferation of marrow stromal cells. One-third patients have a preceding history of PRV or ET.

Clinical features
• Sexes affected equally; age of onset rarely below 50 years.
• Massive splenomegaly may lead to left hypochondrial pain.

• Fever, weight loss, pruritus, hepatomegaly and night sweats are frequent; gout, bone and joint pain are less common.
• Abdominal swelling, ascites and bleeding from oesophageal varices occur, caused by portal hypertension, in late stages.

Laboratory features
• Normochromic normocytic anaemia. This may be severe.
• Leucocytosis and thrombocytosis occur early, and later leucopenia and thrombocytopenia.
• Blood film: red cell poikilocytosis with teardrop forms (Fig. 28.2) circulating red cell and white cell precursors (leucoerythroblastic picture).
• The *JAK2* mutation is present in about 50% of cases.
• Serum lactic dehydrogenase is raised, in distinction to PRV or ET.
• Liver function tests are often abnormal because of extramedullary haemopoiesis.
• Bone marrow aspiration is usually unsuccessful ('dry tap'); the trephine biopsy shows increased cellularity, increased megakaryocytes and fibrosis (Fig. 28.3, 28.4).

Treatment
• Chemotherapy (e.g. hydroxycarbamide) for patients with hypermetabolism and myeloproliferation.
• *JAK2* inhibitors may reduce spleen size and improve symptoms but do not correct anaemia.
• Thalidomide improves marrow function and reduces spleen size in about one-third of cases; trials are in progress with the thalidomide derivative, lenalidomide.
• Supportive therapy with red cell transfusions, folic acid and occasionally platelet transfusions. Iron chelation may be needed.
• Allopurinol to prevent hyperuricaemia and gout.
• Splenectomy or splenic irradiation to reduce symptoms from splenomegaly, anaemia or thrombocytopenia (selected patients).
• Allogeneic stem cell transplantation has cured some younger patients (<60 years).

Prognosis
Median survival is about 5 years; acute leukaemia occurs in about 20%.

Systemic mastocytosis
This is a clonal proliferation of mast cells that accumulate in the liver, spleen, lymph nodes and bone marrow. There is a somatic of mutation of KIT, the stem cell ligand receptor. The disease often presents with urticaria pigmentosa, an itchy erythematous skin rash. Symptoms are related to histamine and prostaglandin release and include flushing, pruritus, abdominal pain and brochospasm. Serum tryptase is raised. Various therapies have been tried.

29.1 The clinical course of chronic lymphocytic leukaemia (CLL). The International (Binet) staging system evaluates enlargement of the following: lymph nodes whether unilateral or bilateral, in the head and neck, axillae and inguinal regions; spleen and liver. Stage A patients are usually asymptomatic and do not require treatment. The peripheral blood lymphocyte count may rise progressively. Stage B patients often require require treatment. Stage C patients require treatment

Stage	A	B	C
Symptoms	No anaemia, no thrombocytopenia, <3 lymphoid areas involved	No anaemia, no thrombocytopenia, >3 lymphoid areas involved	Anaemia, (haemoglobin <10.0 g/dL) thrombocytopenia (platelets <100 x10^9/L)
Treatment	No treatment	e.g. Fludarabine cyclophosphamide + rituximab (FCR) or bendamustine + R or chlorambucil ± R	as B
Med. survival (yrs)	14	7	2.5

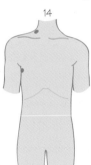
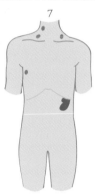
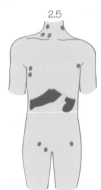

29.2 Chronic lymphocytic leukaemia: peripheral blood film showing large numbers of mature lymphoid cells and some 'smear' cells

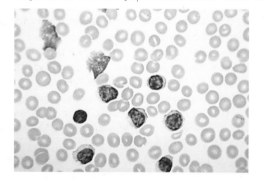

29.3 Hairy cell leukaemia: blood film

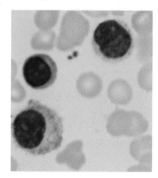

Haematology at a Glance, Fourth Edition. Atul B. Mehta and A. Victor Hoffbrand.

Chronic lymphocytic leukaemia (CLL) is a B-cell clonal lympho-proliferative disease in which lymphocytes accumulate in the blood, bone marrow, lymph nodes and spleen (absolute clonal B lymphocyte count $>5.0 \times 10^9$/L). A disease of older patients (peak age 72 years), it is the most common leukaemia in Western countries (over 70 new cases per million population per year in the UK; male:female ratio 2:1) but is rare in Asia. Small cell lymphocytic lymphoma is an identical disease without lymphocytosis in the blood (see Chapter 33).

Aetiology and pathophysiology

The cause is unknown. The most common chromosome changes are trisomy 12, a 13q deletion and deletions of 11q including the ataxia telangiectasia (*ATM*) gene. Oncogene mutations e.g. of NOTCH1 or deletions occur, which may prevent cells from undergoing apoptosis. The 13q deletion is thought to eliminate expression of several micro-RNAs (see Chapter 20). Mutations or deletions of the P53 gene (chromosome 17) concerned in DNA repair may be present. They have adverse prognostic significance. Mutation of a gene involved in splicing messenger RNA occurs in 15% of cases. This is identical to the mutation found in some cases of myelodysplasia.

Monoclonal B lymphocytosis (MBL) is similar to Stage A CLL but the absolute clonal B lymphocyte count in the blood is $<5.0 \times 10^9$/L. There are no other clinical or laboratory abnormalities. CLL is thought to start as MBL but most cases of MBL do not progress to CLL.

Clinical features

Stage depends on the extent of lymphadenopathy, if present, spleen size and blood count findings (Fig. 29.1).
• Most cases (Stage A) are symptomless and diagnosed on routine blood test. Lymphadenopathy is absent.
• Presenting features in Stage B or C cases include lymphadenopathy (typically symmetrical, painless and discrete), night sweats, loss of weight, symptoms due to bone marrow failure.
• Spleen is often moderately enlarged in Stages B or C.
• Hypogammaglobulinaemia and reduced cell-mediated immunity predispose to bacterial and viral infection e.g. shingles.
• Autoimmune haemolytic anaemia occurs in 15–25% of cases.

Laboratory findings

• Increased peripheral blood lymphocytes (Fig. 29.2; usually $5-30 \times 10^9$/L at presentation) which are B cells (CD19, CD22 but also CD5 positive).
• They have weak expression of surface immunoglobulin M (IgM) which is monoclonal (expressing only κ or only λ light chains).
• Serum immunoglobulins are depressed; a paraprotein may be present in plasma.
• Anaemia and thrombocytopenia may occur due to marrow infiltration, as a result of autoantibodies, or red cell aplasia.
• Expression of a protein kinase ZAP-70 and of CD38 are increased in some (poorer prognostic) cases.
• Degree of somatic mutation in IgH immunoglobulin gene relates to prognosis (Table 29.1). Germline (unmutated) cases are derived from pre-germinal centre B cells (Fig. 31.1) and have a worse prognosis.
• Cytogenetic and molecular changes – these have been described above.

Table 29.1 Prognostic features of chronic lymphocytic leukaemia (CLL)

	Favourable	Unfavourable
Sex	Female	Male
Stage	A	B, C
Lymphocyte doubling time	>1 year	<6 months
Autoimmune haemolytic anaemia	Absent	Present
ZAP-70	Negative	Positive
CD38	Negative	Positive
Somatic mutation at IgH locus	Mutated	Germline
Cytogenetics	13q deletion	P53 deletions

Ig, immunoglobulin

Course and prognosis

Most patients present at an early stage and subsequently remain stationary or progress very slowly. Others present with late-stage disease. Some patients never need treatment, while in others the disease follows an aggressive course. Local lymphoblastic transformation (Richter's syndrome) may occur, with a poor prognosis. The natural history correlates with the maturity of the cell of origin, post-germinal centre (good) or pre-germinal centre (bad) as well as with other clinical and laboratory findings (Table 29.1).

Treatment

• Observation for asymptomatic Stage A patients.
• The purine analogue fludarabine is valuable in combination with cyclophosphamide and rituximab (anti-CD20) (FCR) as initial or subsequent therapy.
• Bendamustine (which has properties both of a purine and alkylating agent) may be used alone or with rituximab.
• Oral chlorambucil gives fewer complete responses than FCR, but is valuable in patients older than 70–75 years.
• Corticosteroids for bone marrow failure due to infiltration and for autoimmune haemolytic anaemia or thrombocytopenia. Typically, the blood lymphocytes count rises initially as lymphocytes are released from tissues, e.g. lymph nodes.
• Ibrutinib inhibits the enzyme Bruton kinase in the B cell receptor signalling pathway in lymphocytes. It is effective in CLL including cases with P53 deletion.
• Alemtuzumab (anti-CD52) may be used in late-stage disease. Careful prophylaxis against bacterial and viral infections is needed. Rituximab is valuable used earlier with chemotherapy. It can also be used to treat autoimmune cytopenias. New anti-CD20 as well as anti-CD22 and CD23 monoclonal antibodies are in clinical trials.
• Support care (see Chapter 21). Immunoglobulin infusions help to protect from bacterial infections, particularly in the winter in profoundly immunodeficient patients.
• Splenectomy or splenic irradiation is useful if the spleen is large, causes local symptoms or hypersplenism and is resistant to chemotherapy.
• Allogeneic stem cell transplantation may cure some younger patients but has a high mortality.

Variants of CLL

Prolymphocytic leukaemia (PLL) resembles CLL but usually occurs in older (>70 years) patients, the white cell count is high and the disease responds poorly to treatment.

Hairy cell leukaemia (HCL) (Fig. 29.3) is rare (male : female ratio of 4 : 1, peak age of 55 years), presents with splenomegaly and pancytopenia. A mutation of an oncogene, *BRAF*, a serine threonine kinase, underlies all cases. 'Hairy cells' are present in bone marrow and blood. They are B cells expressing CD19 and CD20 but also CD11c and CD103. Infections are frequent. Effective treatments include 2-chlorodeoxyadenosine, deoxycoformycin, rituximab, interferon-α and splenectomy.

T-cell variant of PLL is much rarer than the B-cell type and is more aggressive.

Adult T-cell leukaemia/lymphoma is discussed in Chapter 34.

Large granular lymphocyte leukaemia is a rare, chronic clonal disease characterized by a monoclonal T-cell lymphocytosis, often with anaemia or neutropenia. Treatment is usually not needed.

Leukaemia/lymphoma syndromes: circulating lymphoma cells may occur in different non-Hodgkin lymphomas, e.g. follicular lymphoma, mantle cell lymphoma, lymphoplasmacytic lymphoma and adult T-cell leukaemia/lymphoma.

30.1 Multiple myeloma: bone marrow showing infiltration by plasma cells

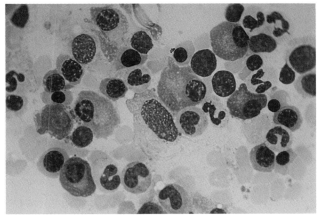

30.2 Multiple myeloma: protein electrophoresis. (a) Lane 22 shows a normal patient. Patient 23 has a paraprotein. The panel on the right shows that this paraprotein reacts with IgG (G) and λ (L) antisera and is therefore of IgG λ type. (b) Data from lane 23 presented graphically and numerically.

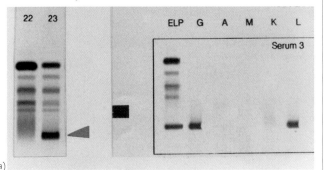

(a)

30.3 Multiple myeloma: skull X-ray showing multiple lytic lesions

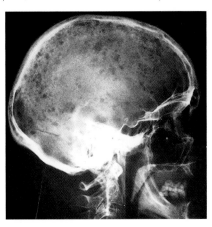

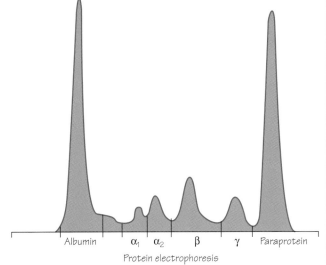

Protein electrophoresis

Name	%	g/L	Normal (g/L)
Albumin	27.2	24.8	35–47
Gammaglobulin	2.1	1.9	25–33
Paraprotein	47.6	43.4	

(b)

Haematology at a Glance, Fourth Edition. Atul B. Mehta and A. Victor Hoffbrand.

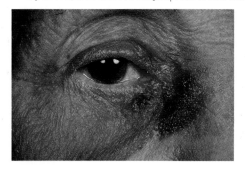

30.5 Amyloidosis: characteristic waxy deposits around the eye

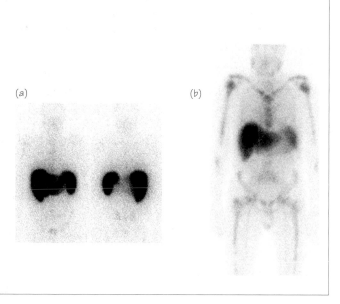

30.6 The P component of amyloid is a normal serum protein designated SAP; it has substantial homology with C-reactive protein (CRP). These patients have undergone a SAP scan – they have been injected with ^{123}I serum amyloid P component (^{123}I-SAP) and then imaged in a gamma camera to identify and monitor amyloid deposits
(a) Patient 1 has extensive deposits in liver and spleen and suffers from systemic amyloidosis (AA) reactive to rheumatoid arthritis
(b) Patient 2 has uptake in bone as well as liver – this pattern is typical of AL amyloid

Multiple myeloma is a malignant disorder of plasma cells characterized by:
1 A monoclonal paraprotein in serum and/or urine;
2 Bone changes leading to pain and pathological fractures; and
3 Excess plasma cells in the bone marrow.

Incidence
Approximately 50 cases per million population; 15% of lymphoid malignancies; 2% of all malignancies; twice as common in black than white people; slightly more common in males than in females; median age at diagnosis 71 years.

Aetiology and pathogenesis
The aetiology is unknown. The cell of origin is probably a post-germinal centre B-lymphoid cell. The cells all secrete the same immunoglobulin (Ig) or Ig component, e.g. part of a heavy chain attached to a light chain or light chain (κ or λ). Rarely (<1%), the cells are non-secretory. Interleukin-6 (IL-6) from myeloma cells themselves or accessory cells promotes plasma cell growth. Tumour necrosis factor and IL-1 mediate bone resorption. Oncogene mutations (e.g. *ras*, p53, *myc*) and translocations to 14q occur. Cyclin D1 is often overexpressed.

Clinical features
• Bone pain, especially lower backache, or pathological fracture due to skeletal involvement.
• Bone marrow failure due to marrow infiltration.
• Infection – lack of normal immunoglobulins (immune paresis) and neutropenia.
• Renal failure occurs in up to one-third patients and is caused by hypercalcaemia, infection, deposition of paraprotein or light chains, uric acid or amyloid.

• Amyloidosis may cause macroglossia, hepatosplenomegaly, cardiac or renal failure, carpal tunnel syndrome and autonomic neuropathy.

Laboratory features
• Anaemia is frequent, often with neutropenia and thrombocytopenia. Erythrocyte sedimentation rate often >100 mm/h.
• Blood film shows rouleaux with a bluish background staining, caused by the protein increase. Leucoerythroblastic picture may be present.
• Bone marrow shows >10% plasma cells, often with multinucleate and other abnormal forms (Fig. 30.1). These cells are CD138$^+$.
• A paraprotein in serum and/or Bence Jones protein (light chains) in urine with suppression of normal serum immunoglobulins is usual (Fig. 30.2a,b).
• The paraprotein is IgG in 70%; IgA in 20%; IgM is uncommon; IgD and IgE are rare.
• Serum light chain (either κ or λ) increased with abnormal light chain ratio.
• Serum β_2 microglobulin (β_2M) often raised and higher levels correlate with worse prognosis.
• X-rays, CT scan or MRI (best for detecting spinal disease) show lytic lesions typically in skull and axial skeleton and/or osteoporosis, often with pathological fractures (Fig. 30.3). Occasional patients show localized plasma cell deposits, typically in the axial skeleton (multiple or solitary plasmacytoma). PET scan can also demonstrate areas of active disease.
• Prognostic data include haemoglobin level, serum levels of β_2M, serum creatinine, serum albumin and extent of skeletal disease. Patients with chromosome 11, 13, 14 and 17 abnormalities have a worse prognosis.

Treatment

• Symptomless ('smouldering') patients who are stable with normal blood counts and renal function, no skeletal disease and low levels of paraprotein warrant observation rather than therapy. High risk patients e.g. IgG paraprotein >30 g/L may benefit from early treatment.

• Chemotherapy is indicated if one or more of C (hypercalcaemia), R (renal failure), A (anaemia) or B (bone lesions) (CRAB) is present. Initial treatment depends on age and performance status. In patients >65 years, induction is usually with melphalan, prednisolone and thalidomide (or lenalidomide). New protocols which include bortezomib (Velcade, a proteosome inhibitor) or lenalidomide (instead of thalidomide) may give improved responses. Both bortezomib and thalidomide may give rise to a peripheral neuropathy as a side effect.

• Most patients will reach a stable (plateau) phase (clinically well with near normal blood count, <5% plasma cells in bone marrow, stable paraprotein level) after 4–6 cycles of treatment. This lasts 1–3 years.

• Younger patients (<65 years) benefit from intensive induction with courses of, for example cyclophosphamide, dexamethasone and thalidomide, followed by high-dose chemotherapy, e.g. with high-dose melphalan and autologous peripheral blood stem cell transplant.

• Most patients relapse and median survival is 5–7 years from diagnosis. Relapsed cases may be retreated with different combinations, e.g. idarubicin and dexamethasone, but may respond again to initial therapy. Derivatives of lenalidomide (e.g. pomalidomide) and of bortezomib (e.g. carfilzomib) are undergoing evaluation.

• Radiotherapy is helpful in relieving pain from localized skeletal disease; hemi-body radiotherapy may help to control systemic disease.

• Allogeneic stem cell transplant may be curative if applied to selected younger (<50 years) patients early in the course of the disease or at first relapse but procedure-related mortality rate is high.

• Supportive care includes hydration to prevent/treat renal failure, allopurinol to prevent hyperuricaemia, hydration, steroids and bisphosphonates for hypercalcaemia, antibiotics and blood components. Bisphosphonates (e.g. oral sodium clodronate, or intravenous pamidronate or zoledronate) are useful in reducing skeletal complications and may improve survival. Surgery may be required for complications (e.g. pathological fracture, spinal cord compression). Plasma exchange is helpful in reducing the paraprotein level quickly. Patients with renal imparment respond particularly well to bortezomib; and those with established renal failure may need dialysis.

Related disorders

Benign monoclonal gammopathy (also termed monoclonal gammopathy of undetermined significance; MGUS) is an indolent disorder, more common than myeloma and characterized by a low (<25 g/L) and stationary serum level of paraprotein, no reduction in normal immunoglobulins, no or mild increase in one or other light chain, absence of skeletal abnormalities and of Bence Jones protein and less than 10% plasma cells in the marrow. It may progress slowly to myeloma in approximately 1% of patients per year of follow-up.

Solitary plasmacytoma may occur in bone or in soft tissues, a low level of serum paraprotein may occur and some cases later develop myeloma.

Plasma cell leukaemia is an aggressive disorder in which large numbers of plasma cells circulate. The prognosis is poor.

Amyloid

Amyloidosis is the tissue deposition of a fibrillary homogeneous eosinophilic protein material which is birefringent and stains with Congo red. It is classified into the following:

• Amyloid derived from clonal lymphocyte or plasma cell proliferation (AL) (e.g. myeloma, primary amyloidosis) when immunoglobulin light chains or components of them are deposited.

• Reactive amyloidosis (AA) which occurs when serum amyloid A protein, an apolipoprotein, is deposited as a result of a chronic inflammatory disease, e.g. rheumatoid arthritis, inflammatory bowel disease or chronic infection, e.g. tuberculosis, leprosy, osteomyelitis and bronchiectasis. Familial Mediterranean fever is a chronic inflammatory disease often affecting the kidneys and joints in which amyloidosis is a frequent complication. It is due to mutation of the pyrinin gene. The protein affects complement activation and neutrophil function.

Localized amyloid occurs in, for example, endocrine organs or skin in old age (Fig. 30.4), with deposition of protein A, hormones and other constituents. There are also a number of rare inherited forms of amyloid due to genetic abnormalities in various proteins.

Amyloid P protein is a serum protein related to C-reactive protein, which is deposited in both AL and AA types of amyloid. Amyloid deposition leads to organ enlargement and dysfunction. Tissues involved include kidneys, heart, skin, tongue, endocrine organs, liver, spleen, gastrointestinal and respiratory tracts and the autonomic nervous system. Diagnosis is made by biopsy of tongue, gums, abdominal fat or rectum with special staining. The extent of the disease can be measured using radioactive-labelled P-protein and whole-body scanning (Fig. 30.5).

31 Lymphoma I: introduction

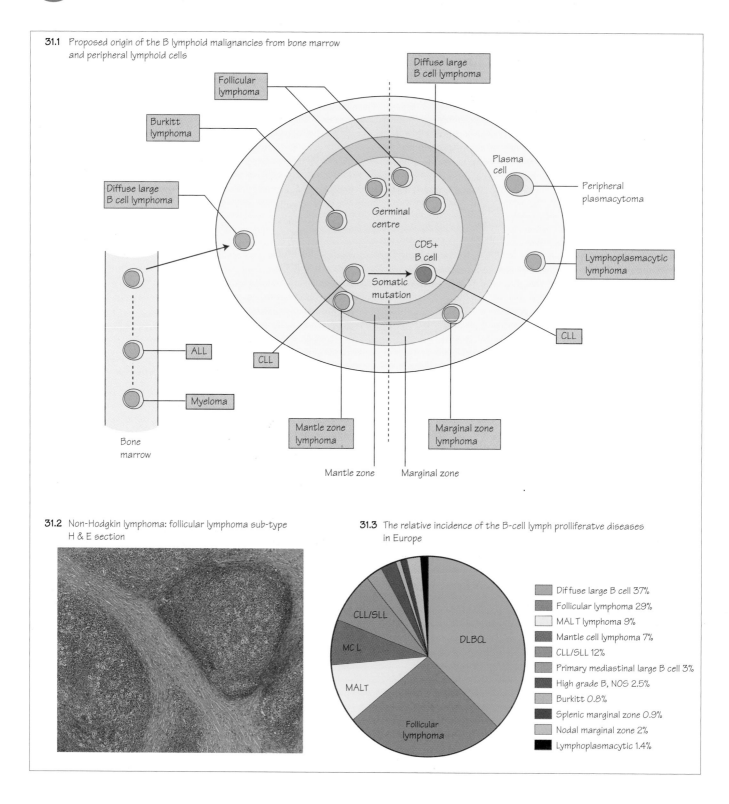

31.1 Proposed origin of the B lymphoid malignancies from bone marrow and peripheral lymphoid cells

Follicular lymphoma

Diffuse large B cell lymphoma

Burkitt lymphoma

Diffuse large B cell lymphoma

Plasma cell

Peripheral plasmacytoma

Germinal centre

CD5+ B cell

Somatic mutation

Lymphoplasmacytic lymphoma

CLL

CLL

Mantle zone lymphoma

Marginal zone lymphoma

Mantle zone

Marginal zone

ALL

CLL

Myeloma

Bone marrow

31.2 Non-Hodgkin lymphoma: follicular lymphoma sub-type H & E section

31.3 The relative incidence of the B-cell lymph prolliferatve diseases in Europe

CLL/SLL

MC L

MALT

Follicular lymphoma

DLBQ

- Diffuse large B cell 37%
- Follicular lymphoma 29%
- MALT lymphoma 9%
- Mantle cell lymphoma 7%
- CLL/SLL 12%
- Primary mediastinal large B cell 3%
- High grade B, NOS 2.5%
- Burkitt 0.8%
- Splenic marginal zone 0.9%
- Nodal marginal zone 2%
- Lymphoplasmacytic 1.4%

Haematology at a Glance, Fourth Edition. Atul B. Mehta and A. Victor Hoffbrand.

Lymphoma is a clonal neoplastic proliferation of lymphoid cells. There are many different types divided into two main groups (Box 31.1): Hodgkin lymphoma (HL) and non-Hodgkin lymphoma (NHL). The NHLs are further subdivided into B-cell diseases (85% of cases) and T-cell diseases (15%) and each of these groups contains many different types.

The lymphomas arise in lymph nodes or in other lymphoid tissue of the body (Fig. 31.1). They are of widely different clinical presentation and clinical course ranging from indolent (low grade) types which may not need treatment for many years, if at all, to aggressive high grade disease which can, without appropriate treatment, cause death within a few weeks of presentation.

The diseases are diagnosed by histological examination of a biopsy specimen, a whole lymph node or, more often, a Tru-Cut biopsy of an affected lymph node. The tissue is stained by the conventional H&E stain (Fig. 31.2) but also by immunohistology using a panel of antibodies conjugated with an enzyme, usually peroxidase. The pattern of antigen expression is determined by visualizing the stained tissue by adding chromogenic substrate to the antibody-enzyme stained tissue. A brown colour indicates a positive reaction (Fig. 20.5). The pattern shows whether the disease is B or T cell in origin; staining for κ or λ light chains can confirm monoclonality of the B cell diseases. In NHL the appearances are often of lymphoid cells, 'frozen' at a particular stage of development. HL is distinguished by the presence of a particular abnormal cell, Reed–Sternberg in the neoplastic tissue (see Chapter 32).

Collectively, the lymphomas are the fifth most common type of malignant disease after lung, breast, colon and prostate cancer in Western countries. NHL is about seven times more common than HL. Its incidence is increasing and it is more common with advancing age. Among NHL, follicular lymphoma and diffuse large B-cell lymphoma are the two most frequent types in Western countries (Fig. 31.5). However, the relative incidence of the various types differs in different parts of the world with, e.g. Burkitt lymphoma being relatively more frequent in Africa and T-cell lymphomas relatively more frequent in the Far East.

The patient usually presents with local or generalized enlargement of the superficial lymph nodes or with systemic symptoms such as loss of weight, fevers, night sweats or symptoms related to a local mass of disease, e.g. in the abdomen, chest, skin or brain. The extent (stage) of the disease is determined by blood and bone marrow tests as well as X-rays, CT scan either alone or with positron emission tomography (PET) scanning (see Fig. 32.4b). The same staging system is used for both HL and NHL (see Fig. 32.3). The spread of the disease tends to form a more regular pattern in HL than in NHL. Treatment in both HL and NHL is partly determined by the stage of the disease.

Box 31.1 The World Health Organization (WHO) 2008 classification (simplified).

Mature B-cell neoplasms
Chronic lymphocytic leukaemia/small lymphocytic lymphoma
B-cell prolymphocytic leukaemia
Splenic marginal zone lymphoma
Hairy cell leukaemia
Lymphoplasmacytic lymphoma/Waldenström macroglobulinaemia
Plasma cell myeloma
Extranodal marginal zone B-cell lymphoma of mucosa-associated lymphoid tissue (MALT-lymphoma)
Nodal marginal zone B-cell lymphoma
Follicular lymphoma
Mantle cell lymphoma
Diffuse large B-cell lymphoma
Burkitt lymphoma/leukaemia
Post-transplant lymphoproliferative disorders. These are usually B-cell and may be polyclonal or clonal (lymphomas)

T-cell and NK-cell neoplasms

Precursor T-cell neoplasms
Precursor T lymphoblastic lymphoma
Blastic NK cell lymphoma

Mature T-cell and NK-cell neoplasms
T-cell prolymphocytic leukaemia
T-cell large granular lymphocytic leukaemia
Aggressive NK-cell leukaemia
Adult T-cell leukaemia/lymphoma
Extranodal NK/T-cell lymphoma, nasal type
Enteropathy-type T-cell lymphoma
Mycosis fungoides
Sézary syndrome
Primary cutaneous anaplastic large cell lymphoma
Peripheral T-cell lymphoma, unspecified
Angioimmunoblastic T-cell lymphoma
Anaplastic large cell lymphoma

CLL, chronic lymphocytic leukaemia; HD, Hodgkin disease; PLL, prolymphocytic leukaemia; SLL, small lymphocytic lymphoma; NK, natural killer

32.1 Hodgkin lymphoma: lymph node biopsy showing (a) Reed–Sternberg (RS) cells (multinucleate cell) (arrows); (b) Immunohistology shows RS cells stain positive for CD30

(a)

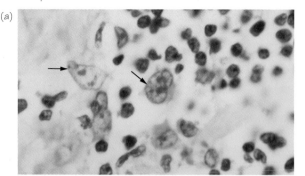

(b)

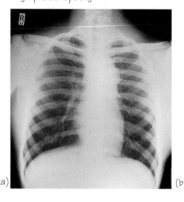

32.2 Hodgkin lymphoma: varicella zoster infection

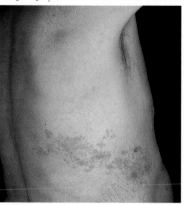

32.4 Hodgkin lymphoma: (a) chest Xray and (b) CT scan showing hilar lymphadenopathy

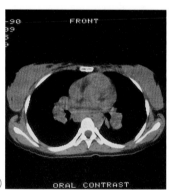

(a)

(b)

ORAL CONTRAST

32.3 Hodgkin lymphoma: clinical features and staging.
Stage I: involvement of a single lymph node region or structure; stage II: involvement of two or more lymph node regions on the same side of the diaphragm; stage III: involvement of lymph node regions or structures on both sides of the diaphragm; stage IV: involvement of other organs, e.g. liver, bone marrow, CNS. A: no symptoms; B: fever, night sweats, weight loss >10% in preceding 6 months; X: bulky disease; >1/3 widening of mediastinum; 10-cm max dimension of nodal mass. E: extralymphoid disease (e.g. in lung, skin)

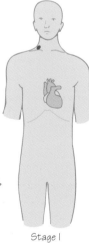 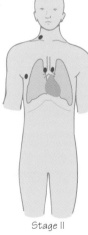 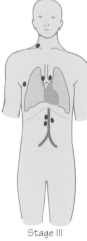 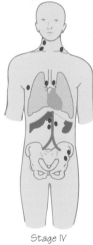

Stage I   Stage II   Stage III   Stage IV

Haematology at a Glance, Fourth Edition. Atul B. Mehta and A. Victor Hoffbrand.

Aetiology and epidemiology

Hodgkin lymphoma is characterized by the presence of Reed–Sternberg cells within the neoplastic tissue (Fig 32.1a). It is more prevalent in males than in females (M:F ratio is 1.5–2.0:1) and has a peak incidence in age range 15–40 years. The cause is not known, but Epstein–Barr virus infection may be a cofactor.

Histological classification

This is well defined and of prognostic significance (Box 32.1). Reed–Sternberg (RS) cells are usually outnumbered by a non-malignant reactive infiltrate of eosinophils, plasma cells, lymphocytes and histiocytes. The RS cells are CD30⁺ (Fig. 32.1b); HL is of B-cell origin. The (classic) disease is classified histologically into mixed cellularity, nodular sclerosis, lymphocyte rich and lymphocyte depleted (Box 32.1). Prognosis for lymphocyte-rich HL is favourable, whereas lymphocyte-depleted HL is less favourable.

Clinical features

- Lymphadenopathy (typically cervical and painless) is the characteristic presentation. The nodes often fluctuate in size, and alcohol ingestion may precipitate pain.
- Hepatic and splenic enlargement may occur.
- Systemic symptoms (fever, weight loss, pruritus and drenching night sweats) occur in 25%.
- Extranodal disease is uncommon but lung, central nervous system, skin and bone involvement may occur.
- Infection caused by defective cell-mediated immunity (Fig. 32.2).

Laboratory features

- Anaemia (normochromic, normocytic; autoimmune haemolytic anaemia can occur).
- Leucocytosis (occasionally eosinophilia).
- Raised erythrocyte sedimentation rate.
- Raised lactate dehydrogenase – useful as prognostic marker and for monitoring response.
- Abnormal liver function tests.

Staging

Staging influences both treatment and prognosis. The most commonly used staging system is the Cotswold classification (Fig. 32.3). Clinical staging with careful physical examination is followed by cervical, thoracic, abdominal and pelvic PET/CT (Fig. 32.4 and 33.2). PET/CT is particularly indicated to exclude distant disease in patients otherwise classified as stage IA or IIA and considered for local radiotherapy. Bone marrow aspirate and trephine are performed to detect marrow involvement.

Treatment

This depends principally on stage and whether or not B symptoms are present.
- Radiotherapy alone is usually used for patients with clinical or pathological stage IA or IIA disease with favourable histology.
- Advanced (stages IB, IIB, III and IV) should be treated with combination chemotherapy (CCT) using one of the standard regimes, e.g. six cycles of adriamycin, bleomycin, vinblastine and dacarbzine (ABVD) or, for more advanced or aggressive disease, or disease not in remission on PET scan after 2 courses of ABVD, escalated treatment.

Local radiotherapy may be needed for sites of bulky or resistant disease.

Relapsed disease

Patients who relapse following radiotherapy alone generally have a very good response to CCT (>80% complete remission (CR) rate). Patients initially treated with chemotherapy who relapse after a remission lasting more than 1 year are likely to achieve CR again and up to 50% may be cured. However, patients relapsing within 1 year of initial therapy, or failing to achieve complete remission, have a poorer prognosis and should be considered for stem cell transplantation (see Chapter 38).

Prognosis

Stage and histology are of importance for HL. While >90% of stage I and II patients may be cured, the rate falls progressively to 50–70% of stage IV patients. Male and older patients generally do less well, as do those with lymphocyte-depleted histology, presentation with anaemia (Hb <105 g/L) or leucocytosis to >15.0 × 10⁹/L (Box 32.2).

33.1 Non-Hodgkin lymphoma: Abdominal CT scan showing multiple enlarged lymph nodes in the paravertebral and mesenteric region

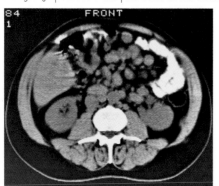

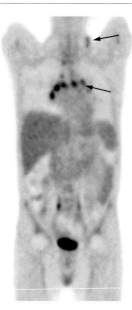

33.2 Positron emission tomography (PET) scan showing persisting areas of active disease in the mediastinum and cervical region (arrows)

33.3 Follicular lymphoma, H and E stain, low power

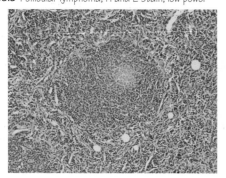

33.4 Diffuse large B cell lymphoma (H and E stain). The architecture of the lymph node is completely effaced by the malignant lymphocytes

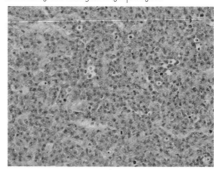

33.5 Diffuse large B cell lymphoma: Immunocytochemistry demonstrates positive staining with the CD20 antibody

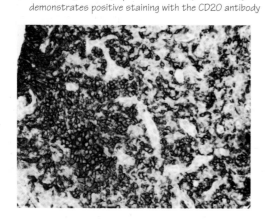

33.6 Diffuse large B cell lymphoma: Immunocytochemistry with the MIB 1 antibody shows positive staining, confirming that nearly all the cells are proliferating

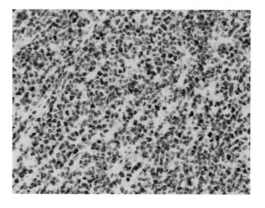

Haematology at a Glance, Fourth Edition. Atul B. Mehta and A. Victor Hoffbrand.

90 © 2014 John Wiley & Sons, Ltd. Published 2014 by John Wiley & Sons, Ltd. Companion Website: www.ataglanceseries.com/haematology

The individual subtypes of B-cell or T-cell NHL are characterized by their clinical and histological features, immunostaining and chromosome changes. The features of some of the more common types are briefly described in Chapter 34. Some of the general features are reviewed here.

Aetiology and epidemiology

Non-Hodgkin lymphoma (NHL) occurs at all ages, with indolent tumours being most common in the elderly. There is clonal expansion from an abnormal cell. Environmental factors relevant to aetiology include abnormal response to viral infection, e.g. Epstein–Barr virus in Burkitt lymphoma (BL); human T-cell leukaemia virus (HTLV-1) in adult T-cell leukaemia lymphoma (ATLL); bacterial infection (e.g. chronic *Helicobactor pylori* infection in gastric lymphoma); and radiation or certain drugs (e.g. phenytoin). Autoimmune disease (e.g. Sjögren syndrome, rheumatoid arthritis) and immune suppression (e.g. HIV infection, post-transplant) also predispose to NHL. Chromosome translocations in NHL involving oncogenes and immunoglobulin genes include t(14;18) in follicular lymphoma (*BCL-2* oncogene), t(8;14) in BL (*MYC* oncogene), and t(11 : 14) in mantle cell lymphoma. A point mutation in *MY88*, a gene involved in the Notch signalling pathway is present in nearly all cases of lymphoplasmacytic lymphoma. Other molecular events may be involved in full malignant transformation.

Clinical features

NHL is heterogeneous, but some common patterns occur.
• Lymphadenopathy is the most frequent clinical feature. It is often widely disseminated at presentation. The lymph nodes may be mainly superficial or deep and detected only by X-ray or scan.
• The spleen and less frequently the liver may be enlarged.
• Extranodal disease is more common than in Hodgkin lymphoma (HL). Involvement of the gastrointestinal tract, liver, central nervous system, skin (especially T-cell lymphomas), lung, thyroid and other organs occurs commonly in the various subtypes.
• Paraproteinaemia is usual in lymphoplasmacytic lymphoma.
• Particularly aggressive lymphomas include BL, some cases of diffuse large B-cell and anaplastic lymphoma, lymphomas associated with HIV infection (often aggressive and intracerebral) and ATLL (see Chapter 34).

Laboratory features

NHL may cause the following.
• Anaemia or pancytopenia as a result of bone marrow involvement leading to bone marrow failure.
• Peripheral blood lymphocytosis caused by the presence of lymphoma cells in the blood.
• Paraprotein (especially in lymphoplasmacytic lymphoma) or hypogammaglobulinaemia.
• Serum lactate dehydrogenase is raised in more aggressive forms.
• Raised serum β_2-microglobulin.

Table 33.1 Immunophenotype of mature B-cell neoplasms

	CD20/19	CD10	CD5	Additional
CLL/small lymphocytic lymphoma	+	−	+	CD200
Hairy cell leukaemia	+	−	−	CD11c CD25c CD103
Lymphoplasmacytic lymphoma	+	−	−	
Marginal zone lymphoma of MALT	+	−	−	
Follicular lymphoma	+	+/−	−	BCL-2
Mantle cell lymphoma	+	−	+	CyclinD-1
Diffuse large B-cell lymphoma	+	+/−	−	
Burkitt lymphoma	+	+	−	

CLL, chronic lymphocytic leukaemia; MALT, mucosa-associated lymphoid tissue

• Cytogenetics by conventional analysis or fluoroescence *in situ* hybridization (FISH) may help to define particular subtypes.
• All patients will require histological diagnosis and immunohistology is essential on Tru-Cut biopsy of a lymph node or bone marrow trephine biopsy to confirm the diagnosis of NHL and define the particular subtype (Table 33.1).

Radiographic features

X-rays, CT scans (Fig. 33.1) and PET/CT scan (Fig. 35.1) are used for initial diagnosis, staging, for monitoring response to therapy (Fig. 33.2) and for detecting low levels of disease when relapse is suspected.

Staging

The staging system is given as for HL (see Fig. 32.3). It is of less importance than in HL, e.g. small lymphocytic lymphoma or follicular lymphoma are often indolent and do not need treatment for many years despite presenting as Stage IV, whereas aggressive Stage I lymphomas may proliferate rapidly locally and require urgent therapy.

Histological classification

NHL is classified as separate disease entities (Box 31.1) based on clinical, biological, cytogenetic, histological and immunological criteria (Table 33.1). Figures 33.3 and 33.4 illustrate the two most frequent types, follicular lymphoma and diffuse large B-cell lymphoma, respectively. Membrane marker and molecular studies of NHL show most (>80%) to be derived from B cells (either follicle centre or from other zones in the lymph node; Fig. 31.2), and the remainder are T cell, natural killer (NK) cell or unclassified. Indolent NHL may evolve into aggressive disease. The proliferation rate of the cells can be assessed by staining for ki-67 (Fig. 33.6).

34.1 Lymphoplasmacytic lymphoma (a) retinal changes of hyperviscosity; (b) improvement after therapy to lower IgM level

(a)

(b)

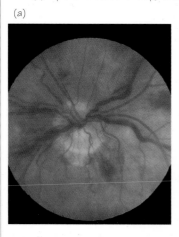
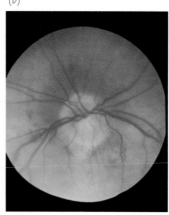

34.2 Spleen enlargement in an elderly female with follicular lymphoma

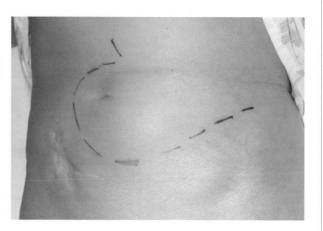

34.3 (a) Lymph node infiltrated by Burkitt lymphoma. Normal nodal architecture is effaced and replaced by large cells, many of which have vacuolated cytoplasm (arrowed)

(a)

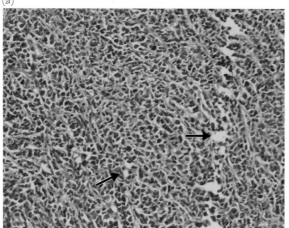

(b) Immunocytochemistry confirms that the cells are of mature B cell lineage (CD 20 positive)

(b)

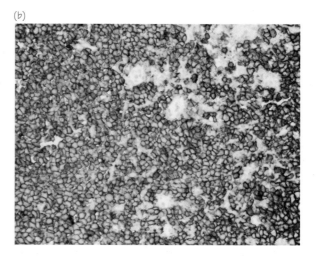

Haematology at a Glance, Fourth Edition. Atul B. Mehta and A. Victor Hoffbrand.

Low-grade B-cell lymphoma

Small lymphocytic lymphoma

This has similar clinical and laboratory features to chronic lymphocytic leukaemia but has no excess of circulating lymphocytes. It is often widespread but indolent and treatment may not be indicated.

Lymphoplasmacytic lymphoma

This is a disease with small lymphocytes, plasma cells and cells with lymphoplasmacytoid appearances in the lymph nodes, spleen and/or bone marrow. There is usually a paraprotein in serum. If this is IgM and >3 g/L, the disease is termed Waldenström macroglobulinaemia. High levels of this protein may be associated with hyperviscosity with visual disturbance, confusion, impaired consciousness and headaches · (Fig. 34.1).

Follicular lymphoma

This is the most frequent form of low-grade lymphoma, mainly involving lymph nodes, usually widespread at diagnosis. The spleen and bone marrow are often involved and the patient may present with a primary skin or small intestinal tumour. The histology is characteristic (Fig. 33.3). It is subdivided into three grades (a–c) depending on the proportion of small and large cells in the neoplastic follicles. Over 80% of cells show the t(14;18) translocation with increased expression of *BCL-2*, which inhibits cell apoptosis.

The clinical course is often indolent for many years with therapy not being needed, but transformation to a more aggressive large cell lymphoma occurs in about one-third of cases when the prognosis is substantially reduced. However, Stage Ia or IIa disease may be cured by local radiotherapy in 50–80% of cases (see Chapter 35).

Marginal cell lymphoma

Splenic marginal cell lymphoma presents with an enlarged spleen, often circulating monoclonal B lymphocytes, autoimmune haemolysis and a paraprotein. Mucosa-associated lymphoid tissue (MALT) lymphomas occur, particularly in the stomach, associated with *Helicobacter pylori* infection in early stages, and this may respond to antibiotic therapy. The disease may also involve the thyroid, lung or other soft tissues.

Mantle cell lymphoma

This usually presents as a low-grade lymphoma with a characteristic histological appearance, small cells with irregular angular nuclei and a diagnostic cytogenetic change t(11;14), which leads to overexpression of cyclin D1. Like chronic lymphocytic leukaemia, CD5 is usually positive. The prognosis is usually poor with a mean survival of only a few years.

High-grade lymphomas

Diffuse large B-cell lymphoma

This constitutes 30–40% of adult non-Hodgkin lymphoma in Western countries. The histological appearances vary but always include diffuse replacement of lymph node structure by sheets of large B cells (Fig. 33.4). Frequently, presentation is extranodal and primary central nervous system disease is frequent in HIV-infected patients. Diffuse large B-cell lymphoma (DLBCL) may arise as transformation of a small cell lymphoma. Despite its aggressive clinical course, DLBCL has a potential to be cured by courses of intensive chemotherapy (see

Table 34.1 High grade non-Hodgkin lymphoma International Prognostic Index (IPI)

	Good prognosis	Adverse prognosis
Age	<60 years	≥60 years
Ann Arbor stage	I or II	III or IV
Serum LDH	Normal	Above normal
Number of extranodal sites	0 or 1	≥2
Performance status	0 or 1	≥2

LDH, lactic dehydrogenase

Chapter 35). The disease may be divided into different prognostic groups by clinical features and serum LDH level (Table 34.1).

Burkitt lymphoma

This is the most aggressive lymphoma which often presents at extranodal sites or as an acute leukaemia. The histology shows a typically 'starry sky' appearance (Fig. 34.3). It occurs in three clinical variants:

1 *Endemic Burkitt lymphoma* (BL) occurs in equatorial Africa and other tropical areas where malaria is frequent. It is common in children and presents with jaw or facial involvement in about 50% of patients with sites including soft tissue organs of the abdomen.

2 *Sporadic BL* occurs throughout the world in both children and adults but accounts for only 1–2% of lymphomas. Patients typically present with abdominal masses, rarely with acute leukaemia.

3 *Immunodeficiency-associated BL* occurs mainly with HIV infection and may be a presenting feature of the infection.

In all types, there is a high risk of central nervous system involvement. Translocation of the oncogene *c-MYC*, usually due to the t(8;14) translocation is present. The individual cells are medium-sized basophilic cells with multiple cytoplasmic vacuoles. Histology gives a starry sky appearance due to pale staining macrophages, which have ingested dying cells, among the high-proliferating tumour cells (Fig. 34.3).

Mature T-cell diseases

These account for only 10–15% of non-Hodgkin lymphomas. They are derived from post-thymic T cells and clinically vary widely from indolent to aggressive tumours with a poor prognosis. The World Health Organization (WHO 2008) lists a large number of sub-varieties, the most frequent of which are included in Box 31.1.

Peripheral T-cell lymphoma, unspecified, is the most common. It is usually nodal, with skin and other extranodal sites frequently involved. Mycosis fungoides (MF) and Sézary syndrome (SS) principally involve the skin; MF without blood involvement shows skin plaques or raised red patches and may become more aggressive with time. SS is more aggressive initially with tumour CD4$^+$ T cells in the blood and lymph node involvement.

Adult T-cell lymphoma/leukaemia occurs in the Caribbean, and other areas where the human T-cell lymphoproliferative virus is endemic. Typically, there is a skin rash, hypercalcaemia, a high white cell count due to leukaemic cells in the blood. Some cases present more as lymphomas with lymphadenopathy or with a chronic course. The neoplastic cells often show polylobated nuclei (flower cells; see also Chapter 29).

35.1 Coronal images (a) pre- and (b) post-chemotherapy for Hodgkin's lymphoma in a 22-year-old male who received treatment on the ABVD protocol. Lymph node enlargement in the mesentery, thorax and axilla has responded to treatment. Axial images from the same patient (c) pre- and (d) post-treatment shows resolution of axillary lymph node enlargement as a result of chemotherapy

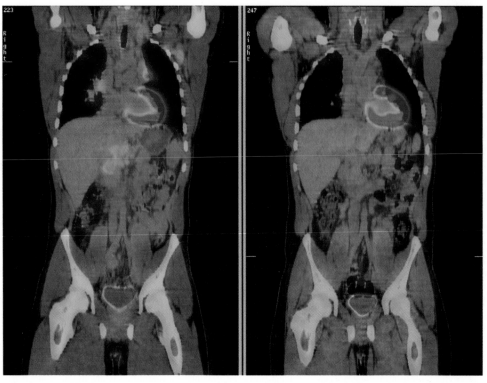

(a)   (b)

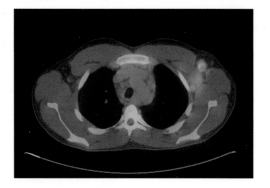 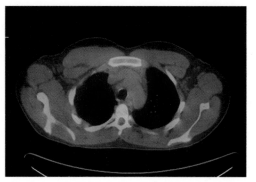

(c)   (d)

Haematology at a Glance, Fourth Edition. Atul B. Mehta and A. Victor Hoffbrand.

94 © 2014 John Wiley & Sons, Ltd. Published 2014 by John Wiley & Sons, Ltd. Companion Website: www.ataglanceseries.com/haematology

Treatment

This depends principally on clinical features, stage and accurate classification by histology including immunohistology and, where appropriate, cytogenetic or molecular studies. Paradoxically, aggressive B-cell tumours respond more dramatically to treatment and are more likely to be cured than indolent tumours. However, they are also rapidly progressive if untreated, frequently relapse and are associated with higher short- to medium-term mortality.

Aggressive

Localized (stage I or II) disease may be treated by deep X-ray therapy (DXT) with adjuvant combination chemotherapy (CCT) (e.g. three cycles of CHOP-R, a 21-day cycle of cyclophosphamide, hydroxydaunorubicin (Adriamycin), vincristine and prednisolone) with anti-CD20 monoclonal antibody (rituximab). Trials are in progress using chemotherapy alone to avoid long-term consequences of DXT. Advanced stage aggressive non-Hodgkin lymphoma (NHL) is treated with CCT (usually CHOP–rituximab, up to complete remission plus at least two cycles); PET and/or CT scan is valuable to assess whether or not full remission has been achieved (Fig. 35.1a,b). DXT to a single site of residual disease may be given.

Diffuse large B-cell lymphoma (DLBCL) may be divided into better or worse prognosis based on immunohistology. More intensive therapy is considered for those with a worse prognosis or who respond poorly to CHOP-R. Patients with central nervous system (CNS) disease are treated with protocols to include high-dose methotrexate and/or cytosine arabinoside aimed at penetrating the blood–brain barrier, with or without CNS radiotherapy. Intrathecal methotrexate therapy is given prophylactically for patients with all forms of aggressive lymphoma with a high risk of CNS disease.

Patients with B or T lymphoblastic lymphoma are treated as for acute lymphoblastic leukaemia (see Chapter 23). Such patients are candidates for allogeneic stem cell transplantation (SCT; see Chapter 38). Patients with Burkitt lymphoma are treated with a different protocol using multiple drugs and incorporating high doses of drugs, e.g. methotrexate and cytosine arabinoside to penetrate the CNS. For HIV-positive patients, treatment of the viral infection with highly active antiretroviral therapy (HAART) is also given.

Relapsed aggressive NHL carries a poor prognosis but may respond to second-line CCT regimes followed by autologous or allogeneic SCT. Treatment of T-cell NHL is similar to that for B-cell tumours except that rituximab is not used.

Indolent

Asymptomatic patients, e.g. follicular lymphoma or small cell lymphocytic lymphoma, may be followed closely without therapy for months or even years. Stage Ia or IIa disease is usually treated with local radiotherapy and may then never relapse. When treatment is required, options include single agent chemotherapy, e.g. chlorambucil or CCT, e.g. cyclophosphamide, vincristine, prednisolone (CVP) with rituximab. Maintenance infusions of rituximab help to prevent relapse. The relapse rate is high. If an indolent tumour transforms to a high grade, intensive therapy is indicated.

Mantle cell lymphoma, despite its similarities to chronic lymphocytic leukaemia and small cell lymphocytic lymphoma, has a poor prognosis and aggressive therapy combined in younger patients with some form of SCT is being tried. *MALT lymphomas* (see Chapter 29) are treated as indolent diseases. Antibiotic therapy to eliminate *Heliobacter pylori* is given in early gastric disease. *Splenic marginal zone lymphoma* responds best to splenectomy.

Mycosis fungoides is treated with skin-targeted therapies, e.g. PUVA, topical steroids, nitrogen mustard or vitamin D. Sézary syndrome is also treated systemically, e.g. CHOP or anti-CD52 (alemtuzumab).

New therapies

Monoclonal antibodies, e.g. alemtuzumab (anti-CD52), anti-CD22, and other monoclonal antibodies, some bound to one or other radioactive toxins, are increasingly used. New CCT regimes have been introduced incorporating fludarabine, bendamustine, mitoxantrone, thalidomide, lenalidomide or pomalidomide, 2-chlorodeoxyadenosine (2-CDA), and bortezomib. Ibrutinib is a promising new agent (see Chapter 29).

Prognosis

Prognosis in NHL is largely dependent on histology. The presence of bulky disease, multiple sites of extranodal involvement, age, performance status and laboratory parameters, such as lactate dehydrogenase level and β_2-microglobulin level, all influence prognosis. Long-term side effects of therapy and supportive care are considered in Chapter 21.

36.1 Aplastic anaemia:
(a) bone marrow aspirate
and (b) trephine biopsy
showing reduced
cellularity with increased
fat spaces

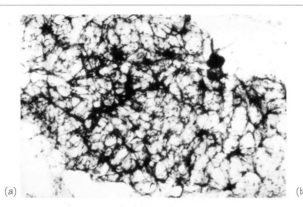

(a)

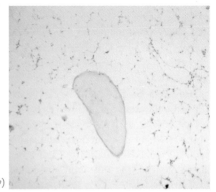

(b)

36.2 Aplastic anaemia: Fanconi's
anaemia, with multiple skeletal
deformities of upper limbs

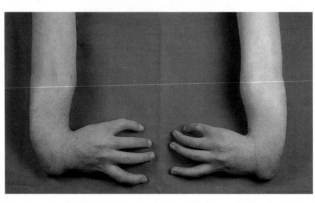

Bone marrow failure

Bone marrow failure is the inability of the bone marrow to produce sufficient red cells, white cells and platelets resulting in pancytopenia (reduction in the blood of red cells, white cells and platelets). Causes are listed in Box 36.1. It occurs most commonly after the administration of chemotherapy and radiotherapy for the treatment of haemopoietic malignancies.

Box 36.1 Bone marrow failure

Primary reduction in haemopoietic cells
Aplastic anaemia
Chemotherapy, radiotherapy

Replacement of marrow by malignant cells
Primary – leukaemia, myeloma, lymphoma
Secondary, e.g. carcinoma

Ineffective haemopoiesis
Myelodysplasia, megaloblastic anaemia

Infiltration by abnormal tissue
Myelofibrosis
Rarely, Gaucher disease, amyloidosis, osteopetrosis

Clinical features

• Symptoms and signs of anaemia, infections and easy bruising or bleeding.
• Symptoms and signs as a result of the underlying cause, e.g. side effects of chemotherapy.

Laboratory findings

• Anaemia, leucopenia and thrombocytopenia of varying severity.
• Blood film typically shows no abnormal cells. It may show circulating red cell and white precursors (leucoerythroblastic) caused by bone marrow infiltration or may show evidence of a primary haematological malignancy, e.g. leukaemia.
• Bone marrow aspirate and trephine biopsy are required to define the cause (Fig. 36.1).

Differential diagnosis

Pancytopenia can also result from accelerated destruction of cells (e.g. as a result of splenomegaly or autoimmune destruction) or pooling of cells (e.g. within an enlarged spleen).

Treatment

• Remove any known cause, e.g. drugs.
• Support care with appropriate blood components and antimicrobials (see Chapters 21 and 49).
• Specific therapy is considered separately with the specific diseases.

Aplastic anaemia

This is a chronic pancytopenia associated with a hypoplastic bone marrow (Fig. 36.1). There are reduced marrow stem cells, increased fat spaces (fat:haemopoiesis ratio >75:25%) and no abnormal cells present.

Aetiology and pathogenesis

The disease may be congenital or acquired (Box 36.2).
- Congenital aplastic anaemia may be inherited as an autosomal recessive (Fanconi type); rarely associated with dyskeratosis congenita (which may be either sex linked or autosomal recessive).
- Acquired aplastic anaemia has an identifiable cause (viral infection, radiation or drug exposure) in about 50% of cases. In the remainder, the cause is unknown but may involve an immune reaction against marrow stem cells.

Clinical features

- May occur at any age, in either sex; incidence of 2–5 cases per million population.
- Onset rapid (over a few days) or slow (over weeks or months).
- Symptoms and signs are caused by bone marrow failure (see above).
- Liver, spleen and lymph nodes are not enlarged.
- Fanconi anaemia usually presents in childhood (Fig. 36.2). Associated findings may include skeletal and renal tract defects, microcephaly and altered skin pigmentation. In dyskeratosis congenita, there are skin, hair and nail changes.

Laboratory findings

- Anaemia is normocytic or mildly macrocytic with a low reticulocyte count.
- Leucopenia is usual with neutrophils below 1.5×10^9/L (<0.2×10^9/L in severe cases).
- Thrombocytopenia (<10×10^9/L in severe cases).

Box 36.2 Causes of aplastic anaemia

Congenital
Fanconi anaemia
Other, e.g. dyskeratosis congenita

Acquired
Idiopathic
Secondary
  Inevitable (cytotoxic drugs, radiation)
  Idiosyncratic
  Drugs, e.g. chloramphenicol, sulfonamides, gold, chlorpromazine, carbimazole
  Chemical agents/toxins, e.g. benzene
  Infection, e.g. viral hepatitis (non-A, non-B, non-C)
Associated with haematological malignancy, e.g. acute lymphoblastic leukaemia
Other, e.g. in association with paroxysmal nocturnal haemoglobinuria

---

- Bone marrow is hypoplastic with >75% fat spaces (Figs 36.1). Remaining haemopoietic cells are of normal appearance. Megakaryocytes are particularly reduced.
- In Fanconi anaemia, lymphocyte chromosomes show random breaks.

Paroxysmal nocturnal haemoglobinuria should be excluded (see Chapter 15).

Specific therapy

- Immunosuppression, e.g. antilymphocyte globulin (ALG), horse or rabbit, given intravenously over several days, and ciclosporin (alone or with ALG) improve marrow function in 50–70% of severe cases. ALG is given with corticosteroids to prevent serum sickness.
- Androgens (e.g. oxymetholone) may benefit Fanconi anaemia and acquired aplastic anaemia.
- Stem cell transplantation offers a cure in severe cases. This requires an HLA matching sibling or unrelated matching volunteer to act as donor. Results are best (60–70% cure) in younger patients (<20 years).
- Haemopoietic growth factors, granulocyte colony-stimulating factor, may raise the neutrophil count temporarily but has no long-term benefit on the underlying bone marrow defect.
- Blood product support (see Chapter 49).

Red cell aplasia

Red cell aplasia is anaemia caused by selective reduction of red cell production by the bone marrow. There is absence or severe reduction of developing erythroblasts in the marrow and of reticulocytes in the peripheral blood, with no abnormality in other cell lines.

Clinical and laboratory features

A rare congenital form (Diamond–Blackfan anaemia, due to a defect in ribosome function) is frequently associated with other somatic malformations. Acquired red cell aplasia may occur as a result of drugs (e.g. azathioprine, isoniazid), in association with autoimmune diseases (e.g. systemic lupus erythematosus), haematological malignancy (e.g. chronic lymphocytic leukaemia) or with a thymoma.

Transient red cell aplasia occurs following infection with B19 parvovirus and can lead to a profound but temporary reduction of red cell production with severe anaemia in patients with a haemolytic disorder (e.g. 'aplastic crisis' in hereditary spherocytosis or sickle cell anaemia).

Treatment

Treatment of the underlying disorder (e.g. removal of a thymoma) is required. Red cell transfusion and iron chelation therapy may be required. Immunosuppressive therapy (e.g. ciclosporin, ALG or rituximab) is useful in selected patients with either congenital or acquired red cell aplasia. Steroid therapy is of questionable value.

Congenital dyserythropoietic anaemias

Congenital dyserythropoietic anaemias are a rare group of recessively inherited conditions in which chronic anaemia results from abnormal maturation of erythroid cells in the marrow. Red cell precursors usually show marked morphological abnormalities, e.g. bi- and trinucleated normoblasts.

37 Haematological effects of drugs

37.1 Drugs may have a wide variety of idiosyncratic side effects on the haemopoietic system (left-hand panel). Side effects of chemotherapy are also given on the right-hand panel and are largely related to the dose/duration of therapy

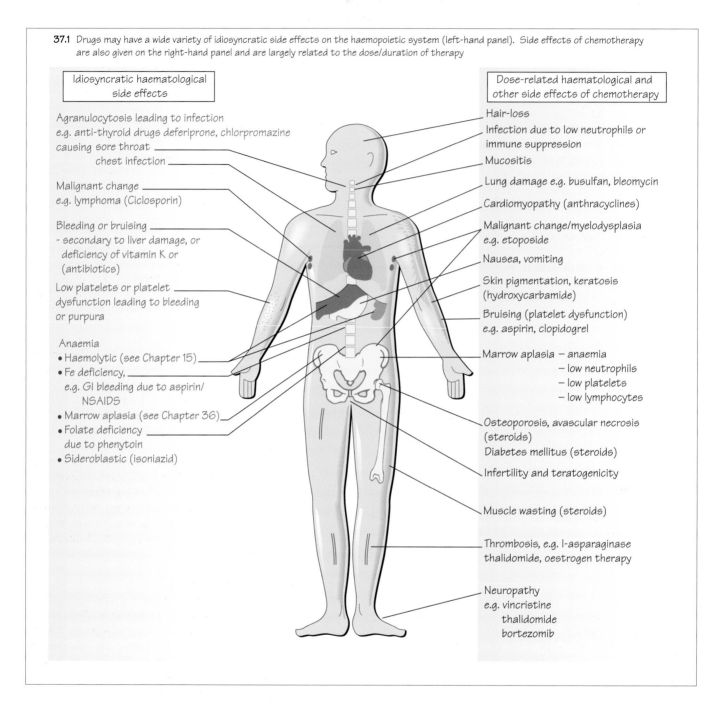

Idiosyncratic haematological side effects

Agranulocytosis leading to infection
e.g. anti-thyroid drugs deferiprone, chlorpromazine
causing sore throat
chest infection

Malignant change
e.g. lymphoma (Ciclosporin)

Bleeding or bruising
- secondary to liver damage, or
deficiency of vitamin K or
(antibiotics)

Low platelets or platelet
dysfunction leading to bleeding
or purpura

Anaemia
- Haemolytic (see Chapter 15)
- Fe deficiency,
  e.g. GI bleeding due to aspirin/
  NSAIDS
- Marrow aplasia (see Chapter 36)
- Folate deficiency
  due to phenytoin
- Sideroblastic (isoniazid)

Dose-related haematological and other side effects of chemotherapy

Hair-loss
Infection due to low neutrophils or
immune suppression
Mucositis
Lung damage e.g. busulfan, bleomycin
Cardiomyopathy (anthracyclines)
Malignant change/myelodysplasia
e.g. etoposide
Nausea, vomiting
Skin pigmentation, keratosis
(hydroxycarbamide)
Bruising (platelet dysfunction)
e.g. aspirin, clopidogrel
Marrow aplasia – anaemia
  – low neutrophils
  – low platelets
  – low lymphocytes
Osteoporosis, avascular necrosis
(steroids)
Diabetes mellitus (steroids)
Infertility and teratogenicity

Muscle wasting (steroids)

Thrombosis, e.g. l-asparaginase
thalidomide, oestrogen therapy

Neuropathy
e.g. vincristine
      thalidomide
      bortezomib

Haematology at a Glance, Fourth Edition. Atul B. Mehta and A. Victor Hoffbrand.

Drugs can cause a wide variety of haematological changes. Two broad categories of effect occur (Fig. 37.1):
• Idiosyncratic – effects that occur only in certain individuals and are independent of the dose.
• Dose-dependent and predictable effects (see Chapters 21 and 36).

Idiosyncratic side effects of drugs

Genetic mechanisms may underlie individual susceptibility to side effects, e.g. G6PD deficiency (see Chapter 14). Genetic traits may also influence drug metabolism, e.g. some individuals metabolize purines so that antipurine drugs, e.g. 6-mercaptopurine, azathioprine, are more likely to cause bone marrow suppression. Others are very sensitive to cyclophosphamide or to warfarin.

Recognizing, monitoring and reporting haematologic toxicity are important parts are of the marketing and post-marketing surveillance and assessment of new drugs. Mechanisms of haematologic toxicity include the following:
• Direct toxicity of the drug or its metabolites to haemopoietic stem cells or more mature cells;
• Induction of immune-mediated damage to haematologic stem cells;
• Effects on folate metabolism;
• Indirect effects via damage to other organs, e.g. the liver; and
• Predisposition to malignant change.

Drug-induced haematological abnormalities

Stem cell damage
• Pancytopenia occurs in a *predictable* dose-dependent fashion following chemotherapy or radiotherapy involving the bone marrow. Chemotherapeutic agents that particularly induce marrow hypocellularity include anthracyclines, epipodophyllotoxins, alkylating agents and antimetabolites.
• *Idiosyncratic* aplastic anaemia occurs rarely (e.g. 1 in 20000–100000 individuals exposed to certain drugs) and is independent of the dose. Drugs with this potential side effect include antibiotics (e.g. chloramphenicol, sulfonamides), antirheumatic drugs (e.g. gold, indomethacin) and chlorpromazine. It is typically severe, up to 50% of patients do not recover their blood counts, and may require treatment for bone marrow failure (see Chapter 36).

Anaemia
The most common form of drug-induced anaemia is iron deficiency due to blood loss. Aspirin, non-steroidal anti-inflammatory drugs (NSAIDs) and corticosteroids can cause bleeding from the upper gastrointestinal tract. Iron absorption is impaired by tetracyclines. Megaloblastic anaemia due to folate deficiency may complicate treatment with antiepilepsy (e.g. phenytoin) and other drugs. Some drugs, e.g.

isoniazid, antagonize vitamin B_6 and cause sideroblastic anaemia by acting as competitive antagonists.

Drug-induced haemolytic anaemias
These may be immune or non-immune. Immune mechanisms include the following:
• Antibody directed against the drug, e.g. penicillin–red cell membrane complex, the drug acting as a hapten.
• Antibody against a drug, e.g. quinidine–plasma protein complex, with subsequent deposition of the immune complex on red cells.
• Stimulation of autoantibody (warm type) production against the red cell, e.g. methyldopa.
   Non-immune mechanisms include the following:
• Haemolysis in G6PD-deficient individuals (many drugs; see Chapter 14).
• Haemolysis in normal individuals, e.g. dapsone.

White cells
Agranulocytosis can occur as part of aplastic anaemia or in isolation. Idiosyncratic agranulocytosis is seen with antithyroid drugs, e.g. carbimazole, deferiprone (0.5–1.0% of all recipients), antipsychotic drugs, e.g. clozapine and antibiotics (sulfonamide, tetracycline). Eosinophilia may be seen as part of an allergic reaction to virtually any drug.

Platelets
Drugs can cause an increased risk of bruising and bleeding by interfering with platelet function, e.g. aspirin and NSAIDs, which inhibit prostaglandin synthesis. Thrombocytopenia may occur as an immune phenomenon, e.g. due to sulfonamides, thiazide diuretics, quinine, alone or as part of aplastic anaemia, e.g. thiazides, sulfonamides.

Coagulation factors
Lowering of coagulation factor concentrations in plasma may lead to increased risk of bleeding, e.g. aspirin-induced hypofibrinogenaemia; or prolonged antibiotic therapy, causing impaired vitamin K absorption. The contraceptive pill (oestrogens) and hormone replacement therapy may cause venous thrombosis because of an increase in coagulation factors and a reduction in circulating levels of coagulation inhibitors, e.g. protein S.

Drug-induced malignant change
Myelodysplasia (MDS) or acute myeloid leukaemia can occur following prolonged use of alkylating agents or combination chemotherapy for acute leukaemia or lymphoma. MDS or non-Hodgkin lymphoma may occur following immunosuppressive therapy, e.g. ciclosporin or azathioprine, which can cause Epstein–Barr virus-associated lymphoproliferative disorders, particularly after transplantation; lymphoma has also been reported following phenytoin therapy.

38 Stem cell transplantation

38.1 Stem cell transplantation. Harvested peripheral blood (PB) or bone marrow (BM) stem cells (SC) may be frozen and stored indefinitely. They may be 'processed', for example to concentrate CD34 cells or remove T cells. Procedures are available to 'purge' them of residual malignant cells (e.g. by use of monoclonal antibodies)

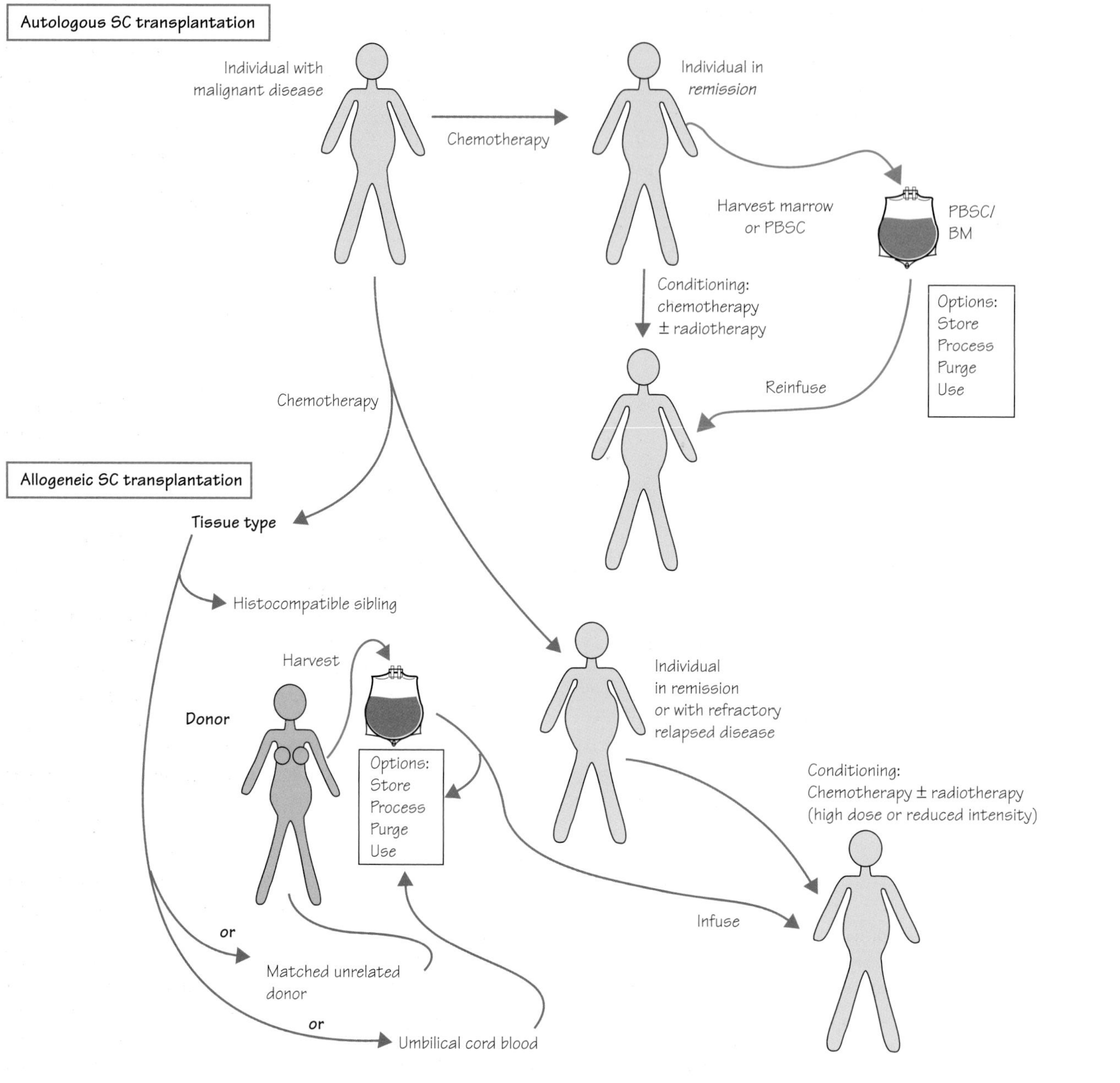

Autologous SC transplantation

Individual with malignant disease

Chemotherapy

Individual in remission

Harvest marrow or PBSC

PBSC/ BM

Conditioning: chemotherapy ± radiotherapy

Options:
Store
Process
Purge
Use

Reinfuse

Allogeneic SC transplantation

Chemotherapy

Tissue type

Histocompatible sibling

Harvest

Donor

Individual in remission or with refractory relapsed disease

Options:
Store
Process
Purge
Use

Conditioning: Chemotherapy ± radiotherapy (high dose or reduced intensity)

or

Matched unrelated donor

or

Umbilical cord blood

Infuse

Haematology at a Glance, Fourth Edition. Atul B. Mehta and A. Victor Hoffbrand.

Stem cell transplantation (SCT) (Fig. 38.1) is the use of haemopoietic stem cells (HSC) from a donor harvested from peripheral blood (peripheral blood stem cells; PBSC) or bone marrow, to repopulate recipient bone marrow.

Allogeneic SCT involves transplantation of HSC from one individual to another. This is usually between two human leucocyte antigen (HLA) matching individuals, most frequently siblings but, in their absence, volunteer HLA-matched unrelated donors (MUD) are increasingly being used. HLA matching includes class I (A, B) and class II (DR) tested by molecular typing. If the donor is an identical twin, the transplant is termed 'syngeneic'. Conventional allogeneic SCT requires the recipient to receive high-dose chemotherapy and often radiotherapy. It is rarely performed in individuals >65 years of age, as it carries risk of treatment-related morbidity and even mortality (up to 5–10%), which increases with age.

Low intensity 'mini' allogeneic transplants are particularly used for older patients (>60 years), because there is less risk of transplant related mortality and morbidity. Less intensive chemotherapy and radiotherapy are used to immunosuppress the recipient. The infused donor stem cells populate the bone marrow and help to completely eliminate the recipient's haemopoietic and immune systems, as well as any residual disease.

Autologous SCT utilizes the patient's own stem cells. These are harvested from the patient and then used to repopulate the marrow after further high-dose chemotherapy and/or radiotherapy. Autologous SCT may be performed more safely in older patients, up to 70 years.

Cord blood transplantation utilizes fetal stem cells harvested at the time of birth from the umbilical cord. It is particularly useful in children. Adults may need two cord blood donations.

Indications

SCT is used in the hope of curing or substantially prolonging remission in patients with a wide variety of haematological and other diseases. Autologous transplants are mainly performed in myeloma after initial chemotherapy or in lymphomas in second or subsequent remission. For allogeneic or autologous SCT, the recipient requires 'conditioning' therapy (chemotherapy ± radiotherapy) pre-transplant to help eradicate malignant disease in the bone marrow and elsewhere and to cause immunosuppression, thereby reducing risk of rejection of donor stem cells in the case of allogeneic SCT. Stem cells (donor or recipient's own) are then infused to rescue the patient from bone marrow

Table 38.1 Conditions for which stem cell transplantation is used

Allogeneic	Autologous
Acute leukaemia (AML and ALL)	Selected patients with:
Chronic or accelerated phase CML	Myeloma
Severe aplastic anaemia	Lymphoma
Myelodysplasia	
Lymphoma	
Myeloma	
Chronic lymphocytic leukaemia	
Thalassaemia major, sickle cell disease	
Severe inherited metabolic diseases, e.g. adenosine deaminase deficiency and Hurler syndrome	

ALL, acute lymphoblastic leukaemia; AML, acute myeloid leukaemia; CML, chronic myeloid leukaemia

failure. The transplanted immune system in an allogeneic SCT may itself have antitumour, e.g. graft versus leukaemia (GVL) effect, and this is the major way in which allogeneic SCT eliminates the malignant disease (Table 38.1).

Procedure

Treatment with a haemopoietic growth factor (e.g. granulocyte colony-stimulating factor), combined in the case of autologous SCT with chemotherapy e.g. high-dose cyclophosphamide, is used to mobilize HSC from bone marrow into peripheral blood, where they are collected by leucapheresis. Alternatively, HSC may be harvested from marrow by multiple bone marrow aspirations, performed under general anaesthesia. Approximately 2×10^8/kg nucleated cells or 2×10^6/kg CD34 cells are needed (CD34 is a surface marker of early haemopoietic stem and progenitor cells). The recipient of an allogeneic transplant then receives immunosuppressive drugs, e.g. ciclosporin and methotrexate to reduce the risk of graft versus host disease (GVHD) (see below).

Initially after the transplant, the recipient is a chimaera with both host and donor cells circulating. In most cases, the circulating blood cells become 100% donor but stable mixed chimaeras may remain indefinitely.

Complications

• Side effects of conditioning chemotherapy/radiotherapy, e.g. bone marrow failure, nausea, alopecia, skin burns, pulmonary toxicity, hepatic veno-occlusive disease, toxicity to endocrine organs, growth retardation and infertility.

• Rejection of transplanted HSC.

• Relapse of original disease. This is sometimes treated by infusion of lymphocytes from the allogeneic donor (donor lymphocyte infusions), which will have a GVL effect.

• Infection following SCT occurs because patients are severely immunosuppressed. Infection may be bacterial, viral, protozoal or fungal. Prophylactic antibiotic, antifungal and antiviral therapy is given. Cytomegalovirus (CMV) negative recipients should receive blood components which are leucodepleted and from CMV-negative donors. CMV infection may cause pneumonitis, diarrhoea, liver dysfunction, skin rash and graft failure, and is a major cause of transplant-related mortality. Ganciclovir and foscarnet are useful in treatment of CMV infection. Prophylaxis against *Pneumocystis carinii* infection is with oral co-trimoxazole and/or nebulized pentamidine.

• Metabolic problems, often caused by multiple intravenous drugs (antibiotics, antivirals, antifungals), renal failure, blood component therapy, intravenous feeding, etc.

• GVHD (allogeneic SCT). Transplanted lymphocytes may recognize the recipient as 'foreign' and mount an immunological onslaught, despite prophylaxis with immunosuppressive drugs and antibodies and cause a skin rash, liver disease and diarrhoea. This acute GVHD (<100 days after SCT) typically begins 7–10 days after transplantation and is graded according to severity. Chronic GVHD (>100 days) presents with a scleroderma-like syndrome with skin, liver, lung, gastrointestinal or joint abnormalities. The incidence of GVHD is higher in older patients. The incidence and severity of GVHD may be decreased by depleting T cells from donor marrow with antibodies, e.g. anti-CD3 or anti-CD52 (Campath)

• Post-transplant lymphoproliferative disease. This is usually a monoclonal B-cell proliferation, often associated with reactivation of Epstein–Barr Virus infection, affecting the gastrointestinal tract, lungs or other organs. It is treated by reducing immunosuppression and treatment as for non-Hodgkin lymphoma.

39 Normal haemostasis I: vessel wall and platelets

39.1 Haemostasis. This requires vasoconstriction, platelet aggregation and fibrin formation (coagulation)

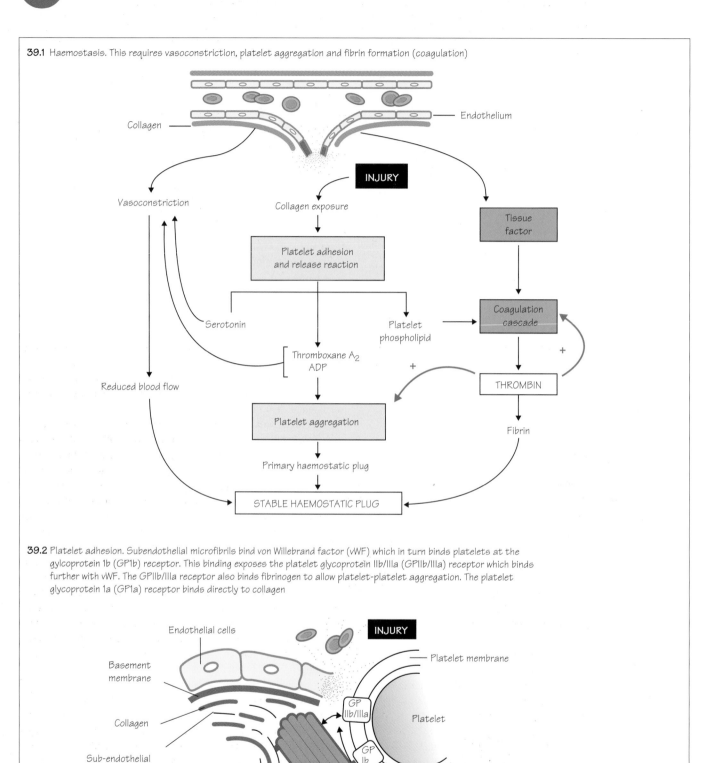

39.2 Platelet adhesion. Subendothelial microfibrils bind von Willebrand factor (vWF) which in turn binds platelets at the gylcoprotein 1b (GP1b) receptor. This binding exposes the platelet glycoprotein IIb/IIIa (GPIIb/IIIa) receptor which binds further with vWF. The GPIIb/IIIa receptor also binds fibrinogen to allow platelet-platelet aggregation. The platelet glycoprotein 1a (GP1a) receptor binds directly to collagen

Haematology at a Glance, Fourth Edition. Atul B. Mehta and A. Victor Hoffbrand.

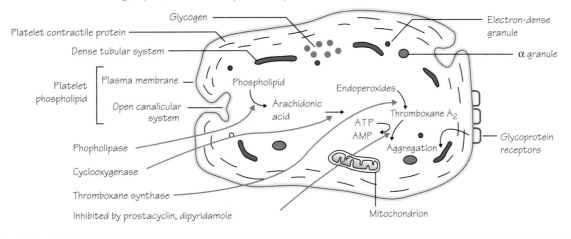

39.3 Diagram of a platelet. Platelets do not have nuclei. Electron dense granules contain platelet nucleotides (ADP), Ca^{2+} and serotonin. α granules contain a heparin antagonist (platelet factor 4), platelet derived growth factor, β thromboglobulin, fibrinogen and other clotting factors. Glycoproteins on the surface, e.g. la (adhesion to collagen), lb (defective in Bernard–Soulier syndrome) and IIb/IIIa (defective in thrombasthenia) are important in adhesion and aggregation. The plasma membrane and canalicular system provides a large reactive surface on which plasma coagulation factors are absorbed and activated. Aspirin and sulphinpyrazone inhibit platelet function by inhibiting cyclo-oxygenase. Prostacyclin from endothelial cells and dipyridamole inhibit the action of thromboxane A_2. Clopidogrel inhibits glycoprotein receptors

Haemostasis is the process whereby haemorrhage following vascular injury is arrested (Fig. 39.1). It depends on closely linked interaction between:
• The vessel wall;
• Platelets and;
• Coagulation factors.

The fibrinolytic system and inhibitors of coagulation ensure coagulation is limited to the site of injury.

The vessel wall

The intact vessel wall has an important role in preventing thrombosis. Endothelial cells produce:
• Prostacyclin, which causes vasodilatation and inhibits platelet aggregation;
• Nitric oxide, which causes vasodilatation and inhibits platelet aggregation;
• Protein C activator (thrombomodulin), which, when bound to protein C, inhibits coagulation (Fig. 40.2);
• Tissue plasminogen activator (TPA), which activates fibrinolysis; and
• Von Willebrand factor (vWF), which can bind platelets (Fig. 39.2).

Injury to the vessel wall: (a) activates membrane bound tissue factor, which initiates coagulation (Fig. 39.1); and (b) exposes subendothelial connective tissue allowing binding of platelets to vWF, a large multimeric protein made by endothelial cells (Fig. 39.2). ADAMTS13 is a plasma protease that cleaves high molecular weight vWF complexes to smaller active molecules. VWF mediates platelet adhesion to endothelium and carries clotting factor VIII in plasma.

Platelets

Platelets are non-nucleated cells required for normal haemostasis. They circulate for 7–10 days. Their lifespan is reduced when there is increased platelet consumption (thrombosis, infection and splenic enlargement). Platelets appear in peripheral blood films as granular basophilic forms with a mean diameter of 1–2 μm. The normal concentration is $140–400 \times 10^9$/L; a lower number is found in neonates $(100–300 \times 10^9$/L) and among certain racial populations, e.g. in southern Europe or the Middle East.

Platelets have a large surface area onto which coagulation factors are adsorbed (Fig. 39.3). Glycoproteins GPIb and IIb/IIIa allow attachment of platelets to vWF (Fig. 39.2) and hence to endothelium. Fibrinogen links platelets to each other by the IIb/IIIa receptor. Collagen exposure and thrombin promote platelet aggregation and the platelet release reaction whereby platelets release their granule contents. Adenosine diphosphate (ADP) promotes platelet activation, aggregation to form a primary haemostatic plug. Platelet prostaglandin synthesis is activated to form thromboxane A_2, which potentiates the platelet release reaction, promotes platelet aggregation and also has vasoconstrictor activity. Platelet activating factor is also released, which further potentiates platelet aggregation. Fibrin, produced by blood coagulation, binds to vWF and enmeshes the platelets to form a stable haemostatic plug. Activated platelets promote coagulation, as they have exposed phospholipid-binding sites which are involved in activation of factor X and prothrombin to thrombin in the coagulation cascade.

Thrombopoiesis (platelet production)

Megakaryocytes are large multinucleated cells derived from haemopoietic stem cells (Fig. 39.4). Platelets break off from the megakaryocyte cytoplasm and enter the peripheral blood. Thrombopoietin (TPO) is produced mainly in the liver and stimulates megakaryocyte and platelet production by increasing differentiation of stem cells into megakaryocytes, increasing megakaryocyte numbers and increasing the number of divisions of megakaryocyte nuclei (ploidy). The level of free TPO in plasma rises when megakaryocte and platelet mass falls and falls when these rise.

Normal haemostasis II: coagulation factors and fibrinolysis

40.1 The coagulation pathway. Injury initiates release of tissue factor (TF) which binds and activates factor VII. The TF VIIa complex activates factors X and IX. The VIIIa–IXa complex amplifies Xa production from X. Thrombin is generated from prothrombin by the action of Xa–Va complex and this leads to fibrin formation. Thrombin also (i) activates FXI leading to increased FIXa production; (ii) cleaves FVIII from its carrier protein vWF activating FVIII; (iii) activates FV to FVa; and (iv) activates FXIII to XIIIa, which stabilizes the fibrin clot

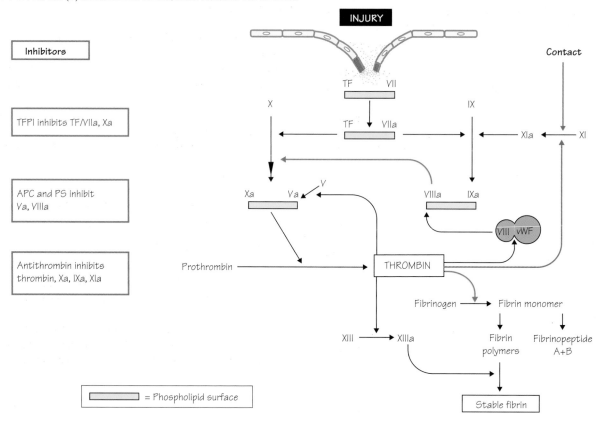

40.2 Fibrinolysis. Injury causes release of TPA and UPA which, together with activated components from coagulation pathway and protein C, activate plasminogen to plasmin. Plasmin acts on insoluble fibrin to form a series of soluble products (fragments)

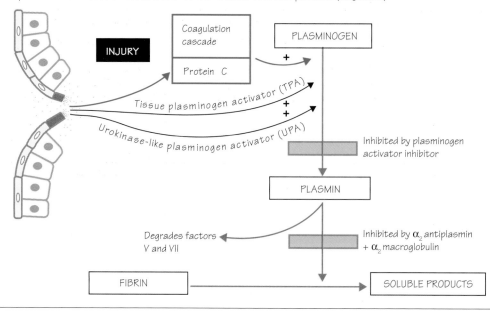

Haematology at a Glance, Fourth Edition. Atul B. Mehta and A. Victor Hoffbrand.

Coagulation factors

The proteins of the coagulation cascade are pro-enzymes (serine proteases) and pro-cofactors, which are activated sequentially (Fig. 40.1). The cascade has been divided on the basis of laboratory tests into intrinsic, extrinsic and common pathways. This division is useful in understanding results of *in vitro* coagulation tests. *In vivo*, however, these pathways are closely interlinked. Coagulation begins *in vivo* when tissue factor is activated on the surface of injured cells and binds and activates factor VII; the complex activates factor X to Xa but also factor IX which, with activated cofactor VIII released from binding to von Willebrand factor (vWF), substantially amplifies activation of factor X to Xa.

The complex of Xa and Va, activated from factor V by thrombin, acts on prothrombin (factor II) to generate thrombin. Thrombin then converts fibrinogen into fibrin monomers, with release of fibrinopeptides A and B. The fibrin monomers combine to form a fibrin polymer clot. Factor XIII cross-links the polymer to form a more stable clot.

Platelets accelerate the coagulation process by providing membrane phospholipids which act as 'docking' stations for the coagulation factors.

Thrombin has a number of key roles in the coagulation process.
1 It converts plasma fibrinogen into fibrin.
2 It amplifies coagulation by (a) activating factor XI which increases IXa production, (b) cleaving factor VIII from its carrier molecule vWF to activate it and augment Xa production by the IXa–VIIIa complex and (c) activating factor V to factor Va.
3 It also activates factor XIII to factor XIIIa, which stabilizes the fibrin clot.
4 It potentiates platelet aggregation.
5 It binds to thrombomodulin on the endothelial cell surface to form a complex that activates protein C, which is involved in inhibiting coagulation.

Coagulation inhibitory factors

These inhibit the coagulation cascade and ensure the action of thrombin is limited to the site of injury.

• Antithrombin inactivates serine proteases, principally factor Xa and thrombin. Heparin activates antithrombin.
• Proteins C and S are vitamin K-dependent proteins made in the liver. Protein C is activated via a thrombin–thrombomodulin complex (Fig. 40.2) and, like protein S, inhibits coagulation by inactivating factors Va and VIIIa; it also enhances fibrinolysis by inactivating the tissue plasmogen activator (TPA) inhibitor (Fig. 40.2).
• Tissue factor pathway inhibitor inhibits the main *in vivo* coagulation pathway by inhibiting factors VIIa and Xa.

The fibrinolytic pathway (Fig. 40.2)

Fibrinolysis is the process whereby fibrin is degraded by plasmin. A circulating pro-enzyme, plasminogen, may be activated to plasmin:
• Following injury, by TPA released from damaged or activated cells; or
• By exogenous agents, e.g. streptokinase, or by therapeutic TPA or urokinase-like plasminogen activator.

Plasmin digests fibrin (or fibrinogen) into fibrin degradation products and also degrades factors V and VII. Free plasmin is inactivated by plasma α_2-antiplasmin and α_2-macroglobulin.

Laboratory tests of coagulation

These are listed in Table 40.1.

Specialized tests

Individual coagulation factors can be assayed by functional tests or immunological methods. Platelet function tests include tests of platelet aggregation with different agonists; platelet function analyser-100 (PFA-100), which measures the length of time blood can be passed through a small orifice before the platelets completely occlude it, and platelet adhesion and assessment of platelet granule contents. Tests for abnormalities leading to thrombosis (thrombophilia) are described in Chapter 44.

Table 40.1 Laboratory tests of coagulation

Screening test (normal range)	Abnormalities indicated (prolonged abnormal)	Most common cause of disorder
PT (10–14 s)	Deficiency/inhibition of factor VII, factors X, V, II and fibrinogen	Liver disease, warfarin therapy, DIC
APTT (30–40 s)	Deficiency/inhibition of one or more of factors XII, X IX, VIII, V, II and fibrinogen	Liver disease, unfractionated heparin therapy, haemophilia A and B, DIC
Thrombin time (14–16 s)	Deficiency or abnormality of fibrinogen; inhibition of thrombin by heparin or FDPs	DIC, heparin therapy, fibrinolysis
Fibrin degradation products (<10 mg/mL)	Accelerated destruction of fibrinogen	DIC
Platelet aggregation tests	Abnormal platelet function	Drugs (e.g. aspirin), uraemia, von Willebrand disease.
PFA-100 test	Platelet functional defect or thrombocytopenia	Drugs (aspirin), von Willebrand disease

APTT, activated partial thromboplastin time; DIC, disseminated intravascular coagulation; FDP, fibrin degradation product; PFA-100, platelet function analyser-100; PT, prothrombin time

41.1 Hereditary haemorrhagic telangiectasia: tongue showing multiple telangiectasia

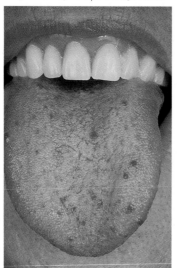

41.2 The forearm of a patient with thrombocytopenia showing bruising at the venepuncture site and small petechial lesions (arrowed)

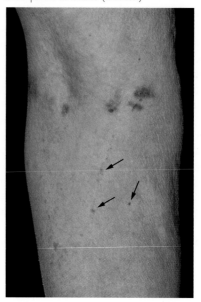

Vessel wall abnormalities

These are associated with easy bruising, purpura and ecchymoses and spontaneous bleeding from mucosal surfaces. Tests of coagulation and platelet function are normal.

Inherited

• Hereditary haemorrhagic telangiectasia is autosomal dominant with multiple dilated microvascular swellings, typically in oropharynx (Fig. 41.1) and gastrointestinal tract, which bleed spontaneously or following minor trauma. Arteriovenous malformations may occur in the lungs or other organs. Local treatment (e.g. nasal packing) may control bleeding; tranexamic acid helps to reduce bleeding. Chronic iron deficiency is frequent.
• Ehlers–Danlos syndrome, Marfan syndrome and other rare connective tissue disorders.

Acquired

Causes include vitamin C deficiency (scurvy), steroid therapy, normal ageing (senile purpura), amyloid in blood vessels, cryoglobulinaemia and immune complex deposition (e.g. purpura fulminans in septicaemia). Henoch–Schönlein purpura is an allergic vasculitis that follows an acute infection, usually in childhood, and may be associated with arthropathy, haematuria and gastrointestinal symptoms.

Platelets

Excessive bleeding caused by thrombocytopenia or disordered platelet function is mucosal (e.g. epistaxis, gastrointestinal bleeding or menorrhagia) or affects the skin (purpura, petechiae and ecchymoses; Figs. 6.1, 6.2, 41.2). Symptoms usually occur when the platelet count is $<10 \times 10^9/L$, but this may be higher when there is impaired platelet

Box 41.1 Causes of thrombocytopenia

Congenital
Rare selective congenital defects of platelet production
Aplastic anaemia (Fanconi)

Acquired
Failure of production
Part of general bone marrow failure
  Bone marrow diseases, e.g. acute leukaemia, myelodysplasia, myeloma, aplastic anaemia, HIV
  Bone marrow infiltration – carcinoma, lymphoma
Cytotoxic drugs

Increased destruction
Autoimmune
Drugs, e.g. heparin
DIC
TTP
Hypersplenism

DIC, disseminated intravascular coagulation; TTP, thrombotic thrombocytopenic purpura

function. Thrombocytopenia (platelets $<140 \times 10^9/L$) may be congenital or acquired (Box 41.1). **Congenital** forms are rare; causes include congenital aplastic anaemia, thrombocytopenia with absent radii syndrome and the Wiskott–Aldrich syndrome (thrombocytopenia with eczema and hypogammaglobulinaemia). Congenital infection (e.g.

Haematology at a Glance, Fourth Edition. Atul B. Mehta and A. Victor Hoffbrand.

106 © 2014 John Wiley & Sons, Ltd. Published 2014 by John Wiley & Sons, Ltd. Companion Website: www.ataglanceseries.com/haematology

rubella, cytomegalovirus) frequently leads to thrombocytopenia. **Acquired** causes include deficient platelet production or accelerated platelet destruction.

Autoimmune thrombocytopenia

The platelets are coated with autoantibody (immunoglobulin) and are prematurely destroyed by the macrophages of the reticuloendothelial system. The acute form usually presents in childhood (2–7 years) and often follows a viral infection. Purpuric rash or epistaxis is frequent. It typically resolves spontaneously. A minority develop mucosal bleeding and should be treated with prednisolone or intravenous immunoglobulin. Up to 20% develop chronic immune thrombocytopenia.

Immune thrombocytopenia in adults is less likely to resolve without therapy and is usually chronic. It is more common in females (male:female ratio is 1:4). Autoantibody is present on the platelet surface and may also be present as free antibody in serum.

Laboratory tests show normal haemoglobin and white cell count; low platelets (often $<20 \times 10^9$/L), normal bone marrow and normal coagulation. Immune thrombocytopenia also occurs in association with some malignancies (e.g. chronic lymphocytic leukaemia, non-Hodgkin lymphoma), infections (e.g. Epstein–Barr virus, HIV, malaria) and connective tissue disease (e.g. systemic lupus erythematosus).

Treatment, if necessary, is with the following:
- Prednisolone (1 mg/kg/day, reducing over 4–6 weeks).
- Intravenous immunoglobulin is valuable for obtaining a temporary rise in platelet count.
- Additional immunosuppressive therapy (e.g. rituximab (anti-CD20), azathioprine, cyclophosphamide, ciclosporin, rhesus anti-D, vincristine) or combination chemotherapy has been used. Danazol (an androgren) is also of value in some cases.
- Synthetic thrombopoietin analogues, eltrombopag (oral) or romiplostim (subcutaneous), raise the platelet count. Prolonged use may cause reversible marrow fibrosis.
- Splenectomy is required for non-responders with continuing symptoms and/or very low platelet counts.

Alloimmune thrombocytopenia

Transplacental passage of antibody from a mother with immune thrombocytopenia can lead to neonatal thrombocytopenia, which typically resolves spontaneously over a few weeks. Mothers who have been sensitized (e.g. by blood transfusion or previous pregnancy) to platelet antigens may develop antibodies which cross the placenta and coat fetal and neonatal platelets, which are then removed in the reticuloendothelial system. Individuals with such platelet alloantibodies can also become thrombocytopenic after blood transfusion (post-transfusion purpura). The antibody is then directed against the HPA1-a antigen on platelets.

Other causes of thrombocytopenia

Drugs cause thrombocytopenia by inhibiting marrow production or by an immune mechanism. The most common immune mechanism (e.g. with quinine, heparin) is when the drug forms an antigen with a plasma protein, an antibody is formed to it, and circulating antigen–antibody complexes are absorbed onto the platelet surface. Heparin-induced thrombocytopenia is associated with thrombosis. A 'heparinoid' drug may be used to continue anticoagulation.

Disseminated intravascular coagulation
See Chapter 43.

Thrombotic thrombocytopenic purpura and haemolytic uraemic syndrome

Thrombotic thrombocytopenic purpura (TTP) and haemolytic uraemic syndrome (HUS) are characterized by thrombosis in small vessels, red cell fragmentation, haemolytic anaemia (see Fig. 42) and thrombocytopenia. Fever, neurological changes and liver dysfunction occur in TTP and renal failure often occurs in HUS. Serum lactate dehydrogenase (LDH) is raised. The prothrombin time (PT) and activated partial thromboplastin time (APTT) are normal.

TTP occurs in adults and may be associated with autoimmune conditions (e.g. systemic lupus erythematosus), pregnancy and infection. It is caused by an acquired deficiency due to an autoantibody to a plasma protease ADAMTS13 which normally cleaves von Willebrand factor (vWF). Abnormally high molecular weight vWF complexes are present in plasma. Congenital TTP is due to lack of ADAMTS13 synthesis.

HUS occurs in childhood and follows infection with verotoxin-producing strains of *Escherichia coli*; or less frequently is associated with *Shigella*, *Salmonella* and streptococcal infection, pregnancy, autoimmune diseases and drugs (e.g. ciclosporin). The ADAMTS13 levels are normal.

Treatment of TTP is with plasma exchange using fresh frozen plasma as the replacement fluid. Antiplatelet drugs (aspirin or dipyridamole), corticosteroids, splenectomy, rituximab and vincristine have all also been used. Response to treatment may be monitored by haemoglobin level, reticulocytes, LDH platelet count, plasma bilirubin and presence of vWF multimers in plasma. In HUS, treatment for fits, hypertension and renal failure are needed.

Disorders of platelet function (Box 41.2)
These are characterized by a normal platelet count, abnormal PFA-100 test and disordered platelet aggregation. **Inherited disorders** are rare and present with bruising/excessive bleeding after surgery or injury in childhood. The most common **acquired** cause is aspirin or other non-steroidal anti-inflammatory drugs.

Box 41.2 Disorders of platelet function

Inherited
Bernard–Soulier syndrome (defective glycoprotein 1b, giant platelets), Glanzmann thrombasthaenia (defective glycoproteins IIb, IIIa), storage pool diseases, von Willebrand disease

Acquired
Drugs: aspirin, other non-steroidal anti-inflammatory agents, clopidogrel, dextran, antibiotics therapy (e.g. cephalosporins)
Myeloproliferative disorders (see Chapters 26–28)
Uraemia
Paraproteinaemia, e.g. myeloma or Waldenström macroglobulinaemia

---

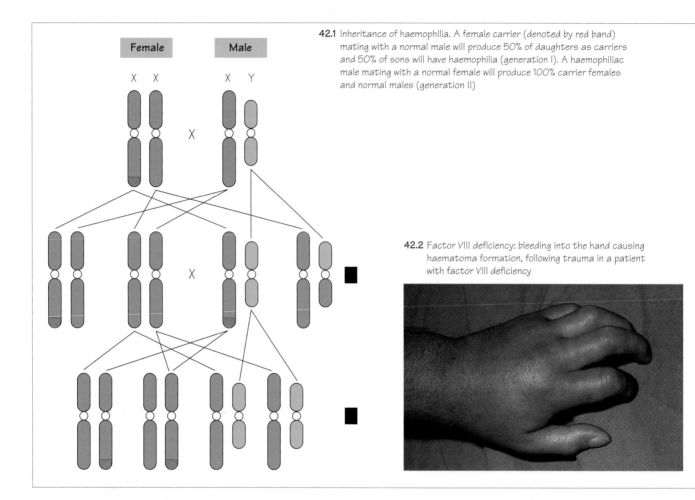

42.1 Inheritance of haemophilia. A female carrier (denoted by red band) mating with a normal male will produce 50% of daughters as carriers and 50% of sons will have haemophilia (generation I). A haemophiliac male mating with a normal female will produce 100% carrier females and normal males (generation II)

42.2 Factor VIII deficiency: bleeding into the hand causing haematoma formation, following trauma in a patient with factor VIII deficiency

Excessive bleeding may occur as a result of an inherited defect of one or other protein involved in coagulation. Inherited deficiency of each of the coagulation factors has been described.

Factor VIII deficiency (haemophilia A)

Factor VIII deficiency (haemophilia A) is the most common inherited coagulation disorder. The factor VIII gene is on the X chromosome so inheritance is sex-linked with the severe disease occurring in males (Fig. 42.1). A wide range of genetic changes of the factor VIII gene including deletions, insertions, point mutations and a common intragene inversion underlie the disease.

Clinical features

• These range from severe spontaneous bleeding, especially into joints (haemarthroses) and muscles, to mild symptoms, depending on the factor VIII level (Fig. 42.2).
• Onset in early childhood (e.g. post-circumcision).
• Increased risk of post-operative or post-traumatic haemorrhage.
• Chronic debilitating joint disease caused by repeated bleeds.
• Pseudotumours as a result of extensive fascial or subperiosteal bleeds.

Laboratory features (Table 42.1)

• Prolonged activated partial thromboplastin time (APTT), normal prothrombin time (PT), normal PFA-100 test. Plasma factor VIII is reduced (<1% of normal in severe cases, 1–5% in moderate cases and 5–40% in mild cases.
• Carriers have factor VIII levels in plasma approximately 50% of normal. If the levels are <40% they may have clinical features of mild haemophilia. DNA analysis is helpful in carrier detection and antenatal diagnosis.
• Von Willebrand factor (vWF) level is normal.

Treatment

• Infusions of factor VIII (either recombinant or concentrate from normal donated plasma) to elevate the patient's level to 20–50% of normal for severe bleeding.
• Level is raised to and maintained at 80–100% for elective surgery.
• Desmopressin, an analogue of vasopressin, leads to a modest rise in endogenous factor VIII which is useful in mild cases.
• Avoid aspirin, other antiplatelet drugs and intramuscular injections.
• Patients should be registered with a recognized Haemophilia Centre and should carry a card with details of their condition.

Haematology at a Glance, Fourth Edition. Atul B. Mehta and A. Victor Hoffbrand.

Table 42.1 Clinical and laboratory features of inherited coagulation disorders

	Haemophilia A	Haemophilia B	von Willebrand disease
Inheritance	Sex-linked	Sex-linked	Dominant
Bleeding	Joints, muscles	Joints, muscles	Mucosal surfaces
PT	N	N	N
APTT	↑	↑	N
Factor VIII	↓	N	↓
Factor IX	N	↓	N
von Willebrand factor	N	N	↓
Platelet aggregation with ristocetin	N	N	↓

APTT, activated partial thromboplastin time; N, normal; PT, prothrombin time

• Patients may need to have continuing or prophylactic treatment at home.
• Carrier detection and antenatal diagnosis can be carried out. New cases due to spontaneous mutations account for about 30% of cases.
• Trials of gene therapy for factor IX and VIII deficiency are giving promising results.

Complications of treatment
• HIV and hepatitis C from impure preparations (prior to the early 1980s), subsequent AIDS, hepatitis and cirrhosis.
• Neutralizing antibodies to factor VIII in 15% of severe patients may require immunosuppressive therapy, treatment with porcine factor VIII, or plasma exchange.

Factor IX deficiency (haemophilia B, Christmas disease)
Factor IX deficiency (haemophilia B, Christmas disease) has similar clinical features to haemophilia A. Also sex-linked, it is four times less common (the gene is four times smaller) and usually milder than haemophilia A. Diagnosis and treatment are similar to haemophilia A, except that factor IX concentrate is used for treatment and desmopressin is not effective. Injection of the gene with a viral vector has resulted in a prolonged rise in plasma factor XI levels in small numbers of patients.

Von Willebrand disease
Von Willebrand disease is usually autosomal dominant and results from mutations in the vWF gene. VWF is a large multimeric protein produced by endothelial cells. VWF carries factor VIII in plasma and mediates platelet adhesion to endothelium (see Chapter 39). The disease is more frequent than haemophilia A; males and females are affected equally.

Clinical features
• Bleeding, typically from mucous membranes (mouth, epistaxes, menorrhagia).
• Excess blood loss following trauma or surgery.
• Haemarthroses and muscle bleeding are rare.

Diagnosis
• APTT is prolonged, PT normal.
• Factor VIII and vWF levels are reduced.
• PFA-100 is prolonged.
• Defective platelet function, reduced aggregation with ristocetin.
• Mild thrombocytopenia may occur.
• The disease is divided into subtypes depending on whether there is a reduction in vWF or different types of functional defect.

Treatment
• Intermediate purity factor VIII concentrate (contains both vWF and factor VIII) for bleeding.
High purity vWF concentrates for severe bleeding.
• Desmopressin is helpful for mild bleeding.
• Fibrinolytic inhibitors (e.g. tranexamic acid) are helpful.
• Carrier detection and antenatal diagnosis based on fetal DNA analysis is available.

Other conditions
Factor XI deficiency is less frequent than haemophilia A (higher incidence among Ashkenazi Jews) and is autosomal recessive. There is poor correlation between factor XI levels and symptoms. It is generally mild, but severe spontaneous and post-surgical bleeding may occur. Congenital deficiencies of factors II, V, VII, X and XIII are rare and usually cause mild bleeding disorders. Factor XII deficiency prolongs the APTT but does not cause clinical symptoms. Fibrinogen deficiency occurs as a moderately severe autosomal recessive disorder. Dysfibrinogenaemia (presence of a functionally abnormal molecule) is both a rare autosomal dominant disorder and a more common acquired disorder (liver disease, malignancy and systemic lupus erythematosus).

43 Disorders of haemostasis III: acquired disorders of coagulation

43.1 Causes and effects of disseminated intravascular coagulation

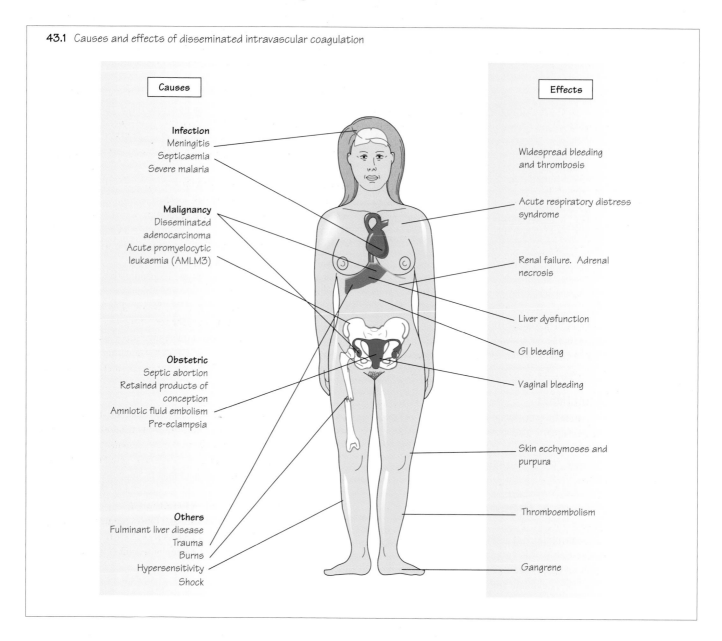

Causes

Infection
Meningitis
Septicaemia
Severe malaria

Malignancy
Disseminated
adenocarcinoma
Acute promyelocytic
leukaemia (AMLM3)

Obstetric
Septic abortion
Retained products of
conception
Amniotic fluid embolism
Pre-eclampsia

Others
Fulminant liver disease
Trauma
Burns
Hypersensitivity
Shock

Effects

Widespread bleeding
and thrombosis

Acute respiratory distress
syndrome

Renal failure. Adrenal
necrosis

Liver dysfunction

GI bleeding

Vaginal bleeding

Skin ecchymoses and
purpura

Thromboembolism

Gangrene

Haematology at a Glance, Fourth Edition. Atul B. Mehta and A. Victor Hoffbrand.
© 2014 John Wiley & Sons, Ltd. Published 2014 by John Wiley & Sons, Ltd. Companion Website: www.ataglanceseries.com/haematology

Liver disease

Liver disease leads to defects of coagulation, platelets and fibrinolysis.
- Reduced synthesis of vitamin K-dependent factors (II, VII, IX, X, proteins C and S) caused by impaired vitamin K absorption (biliary obstruction).
- Impaired synthesis of other coagulation proteins (factors I and V).
- Thrombocytopenia (hypersplenism) and abnormal platelet function (cirrhosis).
- Fibrinolysis impaired.
- Reduced levels of proteins C and S, antithrombin and α_2-antiplasmin lead to susceptibility to disseminated intravascular coagulation (DIC).
- Dysfibrinogenaemia may lead to haemorrhage or thrombosis.

Disseminated intravascular coagulation

Release of procoagulant material into the circulation or endothelial cell damage causes generalized activation of the coagulation and fibrinolytic pathways leading to widespread fibrin deposition in the circulation. The most frequent causes are infections, malignancy and obstetric complications (Fig. 43.1).

Clinical features
- Both bleeding and thrombosis may occur.
- Tissue damage caused by thrombosis leads to necrosis and further activation of coagulation and fibrinolysis.
- Purpura, ecchymoses, gastrointestinal bleeding, bleeding from intravenous sites and following venepuncture may occur as a result of low levels of coagulation factors and platelets resulting from increased consumption.
- Renal function may be impaired due to microvascular thrombosis.
- Other manifestations include acute respiratory distress syndrome (both a cause and a complication of DIC), adrenal necrosis, shock and thromboembolism.

Laboratory features (Table 43.1)
- Thrombocytopenia.
- Nearly all tests of coagulation and fibrinolysis are abnormal with low levels of fibrinogen.
- Fibrin degradation products (e.g. X-DP or FDP) are present in plasma (X = clotting factor).
- Blood film: microangiopathic haemolytic anaemia (see Fig. 15.3) may occur.

Treatment
- Treat the cause, e.g. antibiotics, removal of the procoagulant stimulus (e.g. a dead fetus).
- Supportive therapy with fresh frozen plasma, platelet concentrates and cryoprecipitate if bleeding is dominant.
- Anticoagulant therapy (e.g. heparin) if thrombosis is dominant.
- Protein C concentrate and antithrombin in selected patients.

Other acquired disorders of coagulation

Drugs
- Anticoagulants and drugs affecting anticoagulation (see Chapter 45) are the most common drugs to disturb coagulation.
- Chemotherapy (e.g. L-asparaginase may lead to thrombosis).

Acquired coagulation inhibitors

These antibodies to coagulation factors may be idiopathic, more common in the elderly, or occur in malignancy (e.g. lymphoma), connective tissue disease (e.g. systemic lupus erythematosus) and with paraproteins (e.g. myeloma). They lead to excessive bleeding, both spontaneously and following injury.

Vitamin K deficiency

Vitamin K is required to activate factors II, VII, IX and X and protein C and S by γ-carboxylation (see Chapter 40). It is fat-soluble and derived from vegetables in food and intestinal flora. Deficiency occurs in patients on poor diets, those taking broad-spectrum antibiotics that reduce the gut flora, in biliary tract disease and with intestinal malabsorption.

Massive post-trauma/surgery uncontrollable bleeding

This can be due to multiple factors, DIC with consumption of platelets and clotting factors and excess fibrinolysis. If bleeding persists despite replacement of platelets and clotting factors, recombinant human factor VIIa may be life-saving.

Haemorrhagic disease of the newborn

Newborn infants are at an increased risk of bleeding because of hepatic immaturity and low levels of vitamin K. It is customary to give an injection of vitamin K (1 mg) to all newborn infants in the UK.

Table 43.1 Coagulation changes in acquired disorders of coagulation

	PT	APTT	TT	Platelets	Other
Liver disease	↑	↑	N/↑	↓	Dysfibrinogenaemia
DIC	↑	↑	↑	↓	FDP ↑ ± RBC fragments on blood film
Vitamin K deficiency	↑	↑ or N	N	N	
Massive transfusion	↑	↑	N	↓	
Oral anticoagulants	↑	↑	N	N	
Heparin	↑	↑	↑	N (rarely ↓)	Anti-Xa ↓

APTT, activated partial thromboplastin time; DIC, disseminated intravascular coagulation; FDP, fibrin degradation products; N, normal; PT, prothrombin time; RBC, red blood cell; TT, thrombin time

Thrombosis and antithrombotic therapy

44.1 Transverse ultrasound with colour Doppler of the dilated common femoral vein showing a central filling defect (large arrow) in keeping with thrombus with peripheral flow around the thrombus – shown as red and blue on the colour Doppler. Laterally is a normal common femoral artery showing flow within it on the colour Doppler. Image courtesy of Philips Healthcare

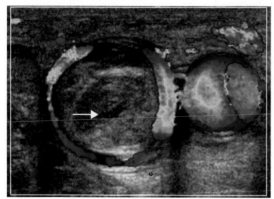

Medial   Lateral

44.2 The protein C pathway. Thrombin bound to thrombomodulin (TM) on intact endothelium activates protein C to activated protein C (APC). This combines with protein S (PS) and inactivates Va and VIIIa. Factor V Leiden is resistant to APC

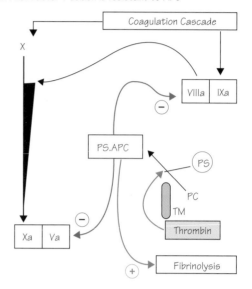

Haematology at a Glance, Fourth Edition. Atul B. Mehta and A. Victor Hoffbrand.

Thrombosis

Thrombosis is the pathological process whereby platelets and fibrin interact with the vessel wall to form a haemostatic plug to cause vascular obstruction. It may be arterial, causing ischaemia, or venous, leading to stasis (Fig. 44.1). The thrombus may be subsequently lysed by fibrinolysis, organized, recanalized or embolized. Thrombosis underlies ischaemic heart, cerebrovascular and peripheral vascular diseases, venous occlusion and pulmonary embolism; it plays an important part in pre-eclampsia.

Arterial thrombosis

This occurs in relation to damaged endothelium, e.g. atherosclerotic plaques. Exposed collagen and released tissue factor cause platelet aggregation and fibrin formation (Box 44.1).

Venous thrombosis

All hospital in-patients are assessed for risk of venous thromboembolism (VTE) and appropriate measures for VTE prophylaxis instituted where indicated. The most common site for deep vein thrombosis (DVT) is the leg which may be below knee or involve veins in the thigh and the iliac veins.

Factors affecting blood flow (e.g. stasis, obesity), alterations in blood constituents and damage to vascular endothelium (e.g. caused by sepsis, surgery or indwelling catheters) are important risk factors (Box 44.2). Diagnosis can be confirmed by imaging, e.g. Doppler ultrasound probe (Fig. 44.1) or, less commonly, venography. Blood tests, e.g. detection of elevated levels of D-dimers, which are derived from fibrinogen, can also be helpful, especially if recurrence is suspected.

Thrombophilia

Thrombophilia is a congenital or acquired predisposition to venous thrombosis. It should be suspected and screened for in patients with thrombosis who are young, have a positive family history, have thrombosis in an unusual site or recurrence and in females with recurrent fetal loss.

Inherited thrombophilia

Inherited genetic mutations may predispose to venous and, more rarely, arterial thrombosis (Boxes 44.1 and 44.2; Fig. 44.2). Presentation with DVT may be during early childhood or in adulthood, e.g. at commencement of oral contraceptives or during pregnancy/puerperium, after surgery or after a long haul flight. Inheritance of a variant form of factor V (factor V Leiden) is the most common (up to 5% of the population). Activated factor V Leiden is more resistant than normal to inactivation by protein C. The risk of thrombosis is increased sevenfold in heterozygotes and 80-fold in homozygotes. Rarer causes include protein C, protein S or antithrombin deficiency or functional abnormality, defective fibrinolysis (see Chapter 42), mutant prothrombin gene and homocystinuria. The combination of two abnormalities often underlies severe cases.

Acquired thrombophilia

Acquired hypercoagulable states are listed in Boxes 44.1 and 44.2. Pathogenesis, e.g. in pregnancy, oral contraceptive pill therapy and malignancy, is multifactorial and relates to elevated levels of procoagulant factors, depressed levels of inhibitor proteins and physical factors (e.g. stasis, surgery).

Lupus anticoagulant (antiphospholipid) syndrome

Despite its name, patients with this syndrome usually present with arterial or venous thrombosis or recurrent miscarriages. It may be associated with systemic lupus erythematosus or other connective tissue disorders, with malignancy or infections or it may be idiopathic. Patients may show a spectrum of antibodies that interfere with phospholipid-dependent coagulation tests *in vitro* and/or react with cardiolipin. The activated partial thromboplastin time (APTT) is prolonged and not corrected by a 50:50 mix of normal plasma with patient plasma. Anticoagulant therapy is needed for patients with thrombosis or to prevent thrombosis in those particularly at risk, e.g. postoperative.

Antiplatelet therapy

The use of heparin and warfarin is discussed in Chapter 45. Antiplatelet drugs and fibrinolytic drugs are discussed here.

• Aspirin (75 mg/day and 300 mg post-myocardial infarction) is most widely used to prevent arterial thrombosis. It inhibits platelet function by inhibiting cyclo-oxygenase, thus reducing thromboxane A_2 production (Fig. 39.3). The combination of aspirin and clopidogrel is used in high-risk cases and for the first year after angioplasty and stent insertion. Aspirin may also reduce the risk of recurrence of DVT after anticoagulation is discontinued.

• Clopidogrel is an adenosine diphosphate (ADP) receptor antagonist. At 75 mg/day it is widely used with aspirin or alone. It is less likely than aspirin to cause gastrointestinal haemorrhage. Prasugrel is a newer drug with a similar action to clopidogrel.

• Dipyridamole (Persantin) is a phosphodiesterase inhibitor which, by raising the platelet cyclic adenosine monophosphate (AMP) levels, reduces their sensitivity to activating stimuli. It is used in patients with prosthetic heart valves and after cardiac by-pass operations.

• Others: monoclonal antibodies directed to platelet glycoproteins (e.g. abciximab, which is directed against glycoprotein IIb/IIIa) or small molecule inhibitors of glycoprotein IIb/IIIa eptifibatide or tirofiban are used, for example, post-angioplasty or stent insertion.

Indications

Prevention of thrombosis in patients with the following:
• Previous myocardial infarction, transient ischaemic attacks and stroke or high risk of first myocardial infarct (acute coronary syndromes)
• Post-coronary artery surgery or angioplasty;
• Severe peripheral vascular disease.
• Thrombocytosis, e.g. myeloproliferative disorders, post-splenectomy; or
• Pre-eclampsia.

Fibrinolytic therapy

This is used to enhance conversion of plasminogen to plasmin (see Chapter 40), which degrades fibrin. It must be used within 5–7 days for venous thrombi or pulmonary emoblus and 5–7 hours for arterial thrombi.

• Streptokinase directly activates plasminogen. Most individuals have antistreptococcal antibodies; a loading dose is therefore required and treatment becomes ineffective after 4–10 days.

• Urokinase has a similar action but may be used if there are high levels of antistreptococcal antibodies. Single-chain urokinase-type plasminogen activator (SCU-PA) has also been developed.

• Acylated plasminogen streptokinase activator complex (APSAC) activates streptokinase bound to plasminogen.

• Recombinant tissue plasminogen activation (TPA) causes activation of fibrin-bound plasminogen only, and is associated with less systemic activation of fibrinolysis.

Indications

• Acute myocardial infarction: streptokinase is usually given with 300 mg aspirin and heparin intravenously.
• Treatment of arterial and venous thrombosis, e.g. pulmonary embolism, peripheral arterial or venous thrombosis.
• In selected patients with acute stroke, after CT scan has confirmed absence of haemorrhage.

Contraindications

Patients with active gastrointestinal bleeding, aortic dissection, head injury or recent (<2 months) neurosurgery and bleeding diathesis.

Side effects

• Bleeding, especially in patients taking anticoagulants or antiplatelet drugs.
• Anaphylactic reactions may occur with streptokinase.

45.1 Heparin binds to antithrombin via a pentasaccharide sequence and induces a conformational change which allows antithrombin to bind Xa and thrombin. The shorter chain length of low-molecular-weight heparin allows binding to only Xa, while unfractionated heparin will bind both Xa and thrombin. Thus, LMW heparin allows a selective inhibition of factor Xa. Modified from Weitz J.I. (1997) Low molecular-weight heparin. *New England Journal of Medicine*, **337**: 688–98

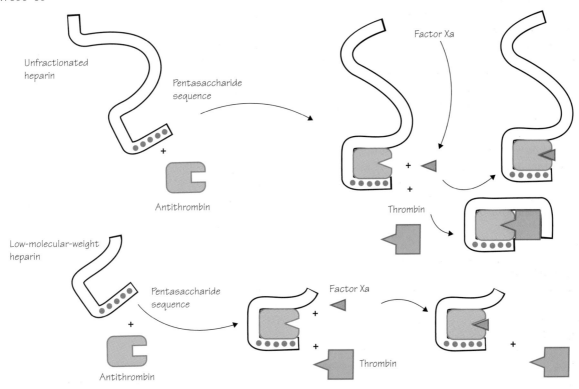

45.2 Action of warfarin

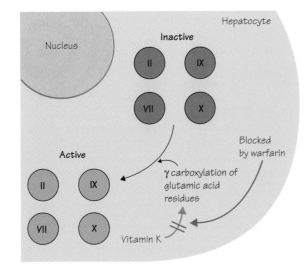

Heparin

Heparin is a mucopolysaccharide that is not absorbed when given orally and is therefore given subcutaneously or intravenously. It activates antithrombin which irreversibly inactivates prothrombin, Xa, IXa and XIa. It also impairs platelet function. Unfractionated heparin (UFH) is a heterogeneous mixture of polysaccharide chains. Low molecular weight (LMW) heparin preparations (MW <5000), e.g. enoxaparin (Clexane), deltaparin (Fragmin) and tinzaparin (Innohep) have a greater ability to inactivate factor Xa and less effect on thrombin (Fig. 45.1) and platelet function, and therefore have a lesser tendency to cause bleeding. They have a longer plasma half-life so that once daily subcutaneous administration is effective in prophylaxis. They also interact less than UFH with endothelium, plasma proteins, macrophages and platelets, making their action more predictable and eliminating the need for monitoring except in certain individuals (see below).

Indications

• Acute venous thrombosis, e.g. deep vein thrombosis (DVT) and pulmonary embolism. Subcutaneous LMW heparin at a therapeutic dose is now usually used. Continuous intravenous UFH can also be given. Warfarin is usually started 2 days after heparin. Heparin can usually be discontinued when international normalized ratio (INR) (see below) is >2.0.
• Unstable angina, post-myocardial infarction.
• Disseminated intravascular coagulation if this is dominated by thrombosis.
• Acute peripheral arterial occlusion.
• Prophylaxis of DVT in surgical and other hospital patients at risk of DVT (LMW heparin once daily).
• Thrombosis prophylaxis in patients undergoing cardiac surgery or renal dialysis.
• Pregnancy. As warfarin is teratogenic, LMW heparin is used in pregnancy when anticoagulation is needed.
• Recurrent fetal loss.
• Maintaining patency of indwelling lines, e.g. Hickman and of catheters.

Monitoring

For continuous intravenous infusion, the activated partial thromboplastin time (APTT) should be maintained at 1.5–2 times normal. LMW heparin therapy is not normally monitored; if necessary, e.g. in renal failure or in those of very low (<50 kg) or high (>80 kg) body weight, it can be monitored by factor Xa assay.

Side effects

• Haemorrhage, particularly if combined with antiplatelet therapy, overdosage or, rarely, platelet function defect. Heparin has a short half-life (1 h); levels fall rapidly when infusion stopped. Protamine sulfate will reverse heparin immediately but must be used with caution as it can cause haemorrhage at high dosage.
• Long-term therapy (>2 months) can lead to osteoporosis.
• Thrombocytopenia, which is antibody mediated. Platelet clumping may cause arterial thrombosis (see Chapter 44).
• LMW heparin is less likely than UFH to cause all these side effects.

Warfarin

Vitamin K promotes the γ-carboxylation of glutamic acid residues of factors II, VII, IX and X; warfarin prevents this. It produces a 50% drop of factor VII levels within 24 hours and of factor II in 4 days. Full anti-coagulation occurs 48–72 hours after starting warfarin therapy. Non-carboxylated factors II, VII, IX and X (proteins formed in vitamin K absence) appear in plasma (Fig. 45.2). Protein C and S levels also fall and this initially (first 2–3 days) leads to an increased risk of thrombosis and may lead to skin necrosis in those with protein C or S deficiency.

The therapeutic dose of warfarin is very variable, ranging from 0.5 to 20 mg/day. This depends on individual variation in its metabolism.

Control of therapy

The prothrombin time is measured and expressed as an INR against the mean normal prothrombin time using a calibrated thromboplastin. Treatment is monitored by maintaining the INR at 2.0–3.0 for most indications, but 2.5–3.5 for those with mechanical heart valves and others at a particularly high risk of venous thrombosis.

Indications

• Treatment of DVT, pulmonary embolism, systemic embolism (3–6-months' therapy).
• Prophylaxis against thrombosis indefinitely in patients with atrial fibrillation, prosthetic valves, arterial grafts, repeated pulmonary embolism and in patients with two or more previous (especially if spontaneous) DVT.
• Low doses (to maintain INR of 1.5) of value in prevention of myocardial infarct in high-risk groups.

Side effects

Haemorrhage – especially in patients taking other anticoagulants, antiplatelet drugs or thrombolytic therapy, and in those with liver disease.

Drug interactions

Warfarin is tightly bound to albumin and is metabolized by the liver. The minor unbound fraction is active. Action is increased by drugs that:
• Reduce its binding to albumin, e.g. aspirin, sulfonamides;
• Inhibit hepatic metabolism, e.g. allopurinol, tricyclic antidepressants, sulfonamides;
• Decrease absorption of vitamin K, e.g. antibiotics, laxatives; and
• Decrease synthesis of vitamin K factors, e.g. high-dose salicylates.
Action is decreased by drugs that:
• Accelerate its metabolism, e.g. barbiturates, rifampicin;
• Enhance synthesis of coagulation factors, e.g. oral contraceptives, hormone replacement therapy.

Reversal of action

Patients with haemorrhage and a raised INR should receive fresh frozen plasma or prothombin concentrates (of factors II, VII, IX and X). If severe, also vitamin K (10 mg intravenously) could be taken, but this results in resistance to warfarin for 2–3 weeks. Raised INR without haemorrhage is managed by withholding therapy for 1–2 days and repeating the INR, but if other risk factors exist, 1–2 mg vitamin K orally should be given.

Other anticoagulant drugs
Direct factor Xa inhibitors

Rivaroxaban is orally active, irreversible and active within 2 hours of administration. It does not need monitoring except in patients with renal failure, children and exceptionally obese individuals. It is given once daily as a fixed dose. It is an effective agent in the prevention and treatment of venous and arterial thrombosis or embolism. Apixaban resembles rivaroxaban in its action but is given twice daily. It is less affected by renal function than dabigatran and rivaroxaban.

Fondaparinux is a synthetic analogue of heparin that inhibits factor Xa selectively. It is given subcutaneously and, like rivaroxaban, does not need monitoring except in specific patients.

Direct factor II (prothrombin) inhibitors

Dabigatran (Pradaxa) is given orally twice daily. Like the factor Xa inhibitors, it acts rapidly and does not need monitoring. It is used at varying doses to prevent venous thromboembolism after orthopaedic surgery, for prevention of stroke and systemic embolism in patients with atrial fibrillation. The dose is varied in elderly patients. Renal function is monitored and the dose reduced or discontinued in severe renal failure.

Reversal of the action of the direct Xa and II inhibitors depends on giving fresh frozen plasma. As their anticoagulant action is short-lived compared to warfarin, patients are not anticoagulated on days they forget to take them.

The identification of thrombin receptors has led to development of receptor antagonist drugs. Hirudin, available as recombinant products lepirudin, bivalirudin and argatroban, is a specific direct inhibitor of thrombin. The preparations are licensed for intravenous use in adults who cannot receive heparin (e.g. because of heparin-induced thrombocytopenia) and also have been used in coronary angioplasty and stenting.

Other treatments

Graduated elastic compression stockings help to prevent DVT postoperatively and to prevent a post-phlebitis syndrome occurring after DVT. Intermittent pneumatic compression of the legs can also be used to reduce the risk of postoperative DVT. An inferior vena cava filter may be inserted to reduce the risk of pulmonary embolus in selected cases if anticoagulation is contraindicated, e.g. ongoing haemorrhage.

46.1 Malaria: peripheral blood film showing red cells invaded by ring forms of *Plasmodium falciparum*

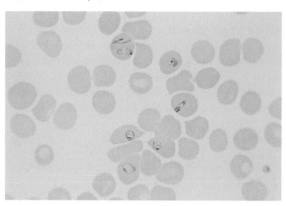

46.2 Malaria life cycle. 1, Sporozoites, injected through the skin by female anopheline mosquito; 2, sporozoites infect hepatocytes; 3, some sporozoites develop into 'hypnozoites' (*Plasmodium vivax* and *P. ovale* only); 4, liver-stage parasite develops; 5–6, tissue schizogony; 7, merozoites are released into the circulation; 8, ring-stage trophozoites in red cells; 9, erythrocytic schizogony; 10, merozoites invade other red cells; 11, some parasites develop into female (macro-) or male (micro gametocytes, taken up by mosquito; 12, mature macrogametocyte and exflagellating microgametes; 13, ookinete penetrates gut wall; 14, development of oocyst; 15, sporozoites penetrate salivary glands

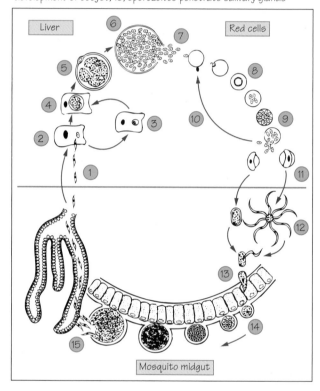

46.3 Leishmaniasis: bone marrow aspirate showing a macrophage containing Leishman–Donovan bodies

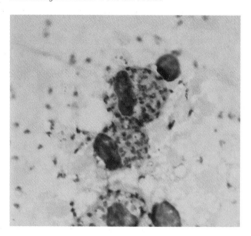

46.4 Trypanosome in peripheral blood

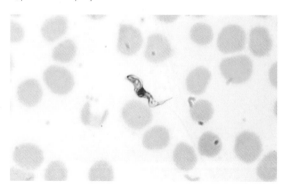

46.5 Jaw tumour in African Burkitt lymphoma

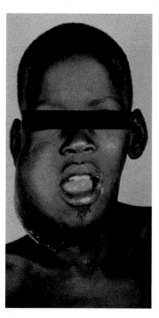

Malaria (Figs 46.1 and 46.2)

Anaemia is caused by haemolysis (cellular disruption and haemoglobin digestion), splenic sequestration, haemodilution (raised plasma volume) and ineffective erythropoiesis. Malarial antigens attached to red cells may cause immune haemolysis. Acute intravascular haemolysis with haemoglobinuria and renal failure (blackwater fever) occurs rarely in *Plasmodium falciparum* infection. Anaemia of chronic disease may also occur. Eosinophilia is variable. Thrombocytopenia occurs in in up to 70% of *P. falciparum* infections and is caused by immune destruction, splenic sequestration and disseminated intravascular coagulation (DIC).

Leishmaniasis

Visceral leishmaniasis is a protozoal infection caused by *Leishmania donovani*. Hepatosplenomegaly, hypergammaglobulinaemia, normochromic anaemia and a raised erythrocyte sedimentation rate (ESR) occur. Bone marrow aspirate shows macrophages containing Leishman–Donovan bodies (Fig. 46.3). Treatment is with pentavalent antimonial compounds or with amphotericin B (AmBisone).

Filariasis

Lymphatic filariasis is usually caused by the filarial worm *Wuchereria bancrofti* and occurs in Africa, Asia and South America. The worms can be over 5 cm long and live in the lymphatics; microfilariae are produced and are seen in peripheral blood smears. The microfilariae are spread from one human host to another by mosquito vectors, and lymphodema (e.g. scrotal oedema) occurs. Eosinophilia is typically quite marked and can lead to acute dyspnoea (tropical oesinophilia). Treatment is with diethylcarbamazine.

Trypanosomiasis

The parasites *Trypanosoma brucei gambiense* (West Africa) and *T. brucei rhodesiense* (East Africa) are transmitted by the tsetse fly. Entry into the bloodstream causes fever, lymphadenopathy, anaemia and splenomegaly. Progressive parasitaemia leads to neurological disturbances including drowsiness and meningoencephalitis. Other complications include haemolytic anaemia, thrombocytopenia and DIC. Diagnosis is by identification of organisms in blood films (Fig. 46.4) from lymph node aspirates. Treatment is with pentamidine and suramin.

Splenomegaly in the Tropics

A number of chronic tropical infections can cause splenomegaly (Box 46.1). The cause is multifactorial and relates to haemolytic anaemia, liver disease with portal hypertension (as in schistosomiasis) and infiltration of lymphatic organs by parasites. The **idiopathic tropical splenomegaly syndrome** is related to previous malaria. Consequences of splenomegaly include abdominal discomfort and pancytopenia. Anaemia is due to haemolysis and an element of dilutional anaemia consequent upon an expanded plasma volume. Thrombocytopenia is due to excessive sequestration of platelets within an enlarged spleen, and leucopenia also results. Bone marrow function is compromised due to parasitic infiltration and an 'anaemia of chronic disorder' occurs. The chronic stimulation of the immune system that occurs in long-standing tropical infection may be a cofactor in the aetiology of lymphoid neoplasia. Thus, the African form of Burkitt lymphoma presents as a jaw tumour in African children (typically boys) and chronic infection with malaria and Epstein–Barr virus are important epidemiological factors (Fig. 46.5).

Anaemia of the tropics

Anaemia commonly occurs in tropical areas and is frequently due to a combination of tropical infection (e.g. haemolytic anaemia in malaria), dilutional anaemia, nutritional deficiencies and anaemia of chronic infection. However, bleeding due to intestinal colonization by hookworm (*Ancylostoma duodenale* and *Necator americanus*) is thought to be the most common cause of iron deficiency worldwide; over 800 million people are thought to be infected. Hookworm infection is also an important cause of prematurity and intrauterine growth retardation. Diagnosis is by identification of the worm eggs in stool. Treament is with benzimidazoles, e.g. mebendazole.

Haematology of pregnancy and infancy

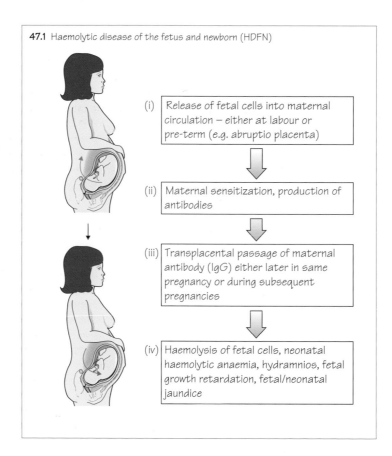

47.1 Haemolytic disease of the fetus and newborn (HDFN)

(i) Release of fetal cells into maternal circulation – either at labour or pre-term (e.g. abruptio placenta)

(ii) Maternal sensitization, production of antibodies

(iii) Transplacental passage of maternal antibody (IgG) either later in same pregnancy or during subsequent pregnancies

(iv) Haemolysis of fetal cells, neonatal haemolytic anaemia, hydramnios, fetal growth retardation, fetal/neonatal jaundice

Anaemia

Plasma volume increases in pregnancy by up to 50% during first and second trimesters, whereas red cell mass (RCM) increases by only 20–30%. Haemodilution results and haemoglobin falls to a mean of 105 g/L between 16 and 40 weeks (Box 47.1). A physiological rise in mean corpuscular volume of 5–10 fl occurs. Increase in RCM, iron transfer to the fetus and blood loss during labour together require about 1000 mg iron, so that iron deficiency is frequent. Folate requirements rise because of increased catabolism. Early supplementation (e.g. 400 μg/day folic acid) reduces risk of megaloblastic anaemia and of fetal neural tube defects (see Chapter 11). The serum B_{12} level falls below normal in 20–30% of pregnant woman, to rise again spontaneously post-delivery. Autoimmune haemolytic anaemia in pregnancy is typically severe and refractory to therapy. Haemolytic anaemia with elevated liver enzymes and low platelets (HELLP syndrome) and epigastric pain may occur in the last trimester. Disseminated intravascular coagulation (DIC) may accompany HELLP syndrome. Induction of labour or caesarean section is often necessary.

White cells

Mild neutrophil leucocytosis with a left shift is frequent.

Platelets

Gestational thrombocytopenia complicates 8–10% of pregnancies, is mild (platelets 80–140 × 10⁹/L) and is not associated with neonatal thrombocytopenia or significant bleeding. Maternal immune thrombocytopenic purpura may antedate or present in pregnancy and is associated with increased levels of platelet-associated immunoglobulin G (IgG) or serum platelet autoantibodies. Management includes careful observation only (absence of bleeding, platelets >50 × 10⁹/L), corticosteroids or intravenous immunoglobulin, which also crosses the placenta to elevate the fetal platelet count. Thrombocytopenia occurs in pre-eclampsia (mechanism unknown); low-dose aspirin therapy may be helpful and may reduce platelet consumption.

Coagulation changes

Coagulation changes (Box 47.1) combine to give an increased risk of thrombosis and DIC. This occurs in up to 40% of cases of abruptio placenta. Retention of a dead fetus usually leads to chronic low-grade DIC with onset over 1–2 weeks. Venous stasis resulting from the gravid uterus combines with increasing clotting proteins to make pregnancy a hypercoagulable state; operative delivery imposes an additional risk of post-partum DVT.

Haemolytic disease of the fetus and newborn

Haemolytic disease of the fetus and newborn (HDFN) is the haemolysis of fetal or neonatal red cells caused by transplacental passage of maternal red cell antibodies (Fig. 47.1).

Haematology at a Glance, Fourth Edition. Atul B. Mehta and A. Victor Hoffbrand.

HDFN caused by ABO antibodies

Although ABO incompatibility between mother and fetus is common, this type of HDFN is rarely severe. Most ABO antibodies are IgM and therefore cannot cross the placenta. Fetal A and B antigens are not fully developed at birth, and the maternal IgG antibodies that do cross the placenta can be partially neutralized by A and B antigens present on other cells, in the plasma and in the tissue fluids.

HDFN caused by Rh and other antibodies

The most important cause is anti-D, produced in Rh(D)-negative woman as a result of sensitization during a previous miscarriage, pregnancy or blood transfusion and causing haemolysis in Rh(D)-positive infants. Other important causes are other antibodies within the Rh system, e.g. anti-C; anti-Kell, anti-Duffy and anti-JKa antibodies may also rarely cause HDFN.

Haemolysis of fetal cells can lead to hydrops foetalis, although nowadays it more commonly leads to neonatal haemolytic anaemia. All women must have their blood group determined at booking and atypical red cell antibodies in plasma should be sought. If present, their titre is monitored throughout pregnancy. Ultrasound for fetal growth, fetal blood sampling and measurements of bilirubin levels in amniotic fluid are used to monitor fetal well-being.

Treatment

Fetuses may be given transfusion of fresh red cells (cytomegalovirus-negative, irradiated) compatible with maternal serum. Maternal antibody levels can be lowered by plasma exchange. Phototherapy and exchange transfusion of the neonate allow removal of unconjugated bilirubin, which may otherwise deposit in the basal ganglia to cause neurological sequelae (kernicterus).

Prevention

This is by administration of anti-D to unsensitized Rh(D)-negative women within 72 hours of a potentially sensitizing event (e.g. birth of an Rh(D)-positive fetus, abortion or antepartum haemorrhage). The anti-D will coat fetal cells which are then removed from the maternal circulation before sensitization occurs. The dose of anti-D is adjusted according to the number of fetal cells detected in the maternal circulation (Kleihauer test or by flow cytometry).

Neonatal haematology

Anaemia – normal neonates have a raised Hb (160–185 g/L). Premature infants are typically anaemic, and this worsens over the course of the first 6 weeks. Deficiency of iron, vitamin E and folate may contribute. Neonates (particularly premature) have an increased susceptibility to infection, although typically have normal leucocyte counts. Important causes of neonatal thrombocytopenia are congenital infection (e.g. maternal cytomegalovirus, rubella and toxoplasmosis) and neonatal alloimmune thrombocytopenia (due to transplacental passage of anti-HPA-1a, antibodies).

Haemorrhagic disease of the newborn is discussed in Chapter 43.

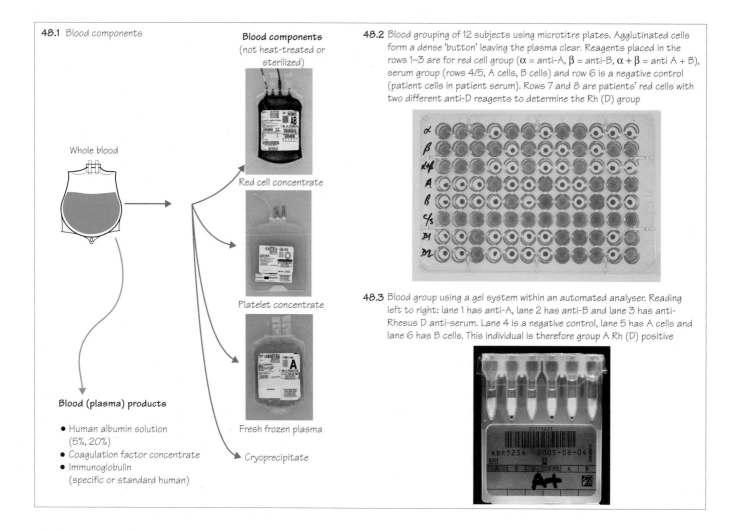

48.1 Blood components

Whole blood

Blood components
(not heat-treated or sterilized)

Red cell concentrate

Platelet concentrate

Fresh frozen plasma

Cryoprecipitate

Blood (plasma) products

- Human albumin solution (5%, 20%)
- Coagulation factor concentrate
- Immunoglobulin (specific or standard human)

48.2 Blood grouping of 12 subjects using microtitre plates. Agglutinated cells form a dense 'button' leaving the plasma clear. Reagents placed in the rows 1–3 are for red cell group (α = anti-A, β = anti-B, α + β = anti A + B), serum group (rows 4/5, A cells, B cells) and row 6 is a negative control (patient cells in patient serum). Rows 7 and 8 are patients' red cells with two different anti-D reagents to determine the Rh (D) group

48.3 Blood group using a gel system within an automated analyser. Reading left to right: lane 1 has anti-A, lane 2 has anti-B and lane 3 has anti-Rhesus D anti-serum. Lane 4 is a negative control, lane 5 has A cells and lane 6 has B cells. This individual is therefore group A Rh (D) positive

Whole blood or plasma is collected from volunteer donors. Over 90% of the donated blood is separated to allow use of individual cell components and plasma from which specific blood products can be manufactured (Fig. 48.1).

In the UK, blood donors are healthy volunteers, aged 17–70 years, who are not on medication, have had no serious previous illnesses and are at low risk for transmitting infectious agents. Those who have received blood product transfusions, drug abusers, haemophiliacs, selected individuals who have recently travelled outside Europe or lived in Africa – where malaria or AIDS may be endemic – and their sexual partners are excluded. Donors are screened for anaemia and they donate two to three times each year.

Donated blood is routinely tested in the UK:
- For hepatitis B and C, HIV 1 and 2, HTLV I and II, *Treponema pallidum*;
- Serologically to determine the blood group (A, B or O) and Rh C, D and E type;
- Selective testing for antibodies to cytomegalovirus (CMV) is used to identify donations which are CMV-negative and thus suitable for certain patients; and

- In other parts of the world, testing is performed for trypanosomiasis (Chagas disease) or West Nile virus.

Blood grouping and compatibility testing
Red cells
Red cells have surface antigens which are glycoproteins or glycolipids (Table 48.1). Individuals lacking a red cell antigen may make alloantibodies (antibodies in one individual reacting to cells of another individual) if exposed to it by transfusion or by transfer of fetal red cells across the placenta in pregnancy. Antibodies to ABO antigens occur naturally, are IgM and complete (detectable by incubation of red cells with antibody in saline at room temperature). Antibodies to other red cell antigens appear only after sensitization. They are usually IgG and incomplete, detected by special techniques, e.g. enzyme-treated red cells, addition of albumin to the reaction mixture or the indirect antiglobulin reaction. Alloantibodies can cause:
- intravascular (e.g. ABO incompatibility) or extravascular (e.g. Rh incompatibility) haemolysis of donor red cells in the recipient; and
- haemolytic disease of the fetus and newborn because of transplacental passage.

Haematology at a Glance, Fourth Edition. Atul B. Mehta and A. Victor Hoffbrand.

Table 48.1 Red cell antigens and antibodies. Incidence in UK individuals given in brackets

Cell antigens	Naturally occurring antibodies (usually IgM)	Antibodies only occurring after sensitization ('atypical' or immune (usually IgG)
A (40%)	Anti-B	
B (8%)	Anti-A	
AB (3%)	–	
O (45%)	Anti-A and anti-B	
Rh (D) (85%)	–	
Rh cde/cde (i.e. Rh-negative) (15%)	–	Anti-D (anti-C, anti-c, anti-E less common)
Kell (K) (9%)	–	Anti-Kell
Duffy (Fya, Fyb) (60%)	–	Anti-Duffy
Kidd (JKa, JKb) (75%)	–	Anti-Kidd

NB: red cells with antigens AA or AO group as A; BB or BO group as B; DD or Dd as D

Blood grouping

An individual's red cell group is determined by suspending washed red cells with diluted anti-A, anti-B, anti-AB and anti-Rh(D). This is usually carried out in microtitre plates (Fig. 48.2) or gels (Fig. 48.3), but automated machines are increasingly used. Agglutination indicates a positive test. Serum is simultaneously incubated with group A, B and O cells to confirm the presence of the expected naturally occurring ABO antibodies. The recipient's serum is also incubated against a pool of group O cells which together express the most common antigens against which 'atypical' antibodies occur. If such an antibody is found, it is characterized and donor blood negative for the corresponding antigen is used for transfusion.

Compatibility testing

Compatibility testing (cross-matching) entails suspension of red cells from a donor pack with recipient serum, incubation (at room temperature and 37°C) to allow reactions to occur and examination for agglutination, including indirect antiglobulin test to ensure that no reaction has occurred.

Red cell transfusion

Indications

• Haemorrhage – if severe e.g. during surgery, post-trauma, post-partum, gastro-intestinal
• Severe anaemia refractory to other therapy or needing rapid correction.

• If repeated transfusions likely, phenotyped ABO and Rh(D) compatible red cells that correspond as closely as possible to the minor red cell antigens of the recipient are used to minimize sensitization.

Types of red cells

• Fresh whole blood (<5 days post-collection) is preferable for neonates.
• Red cells ('packed') in optimal additive solution, e.g. containing sodium chloride, adenine, glucose and mannitol (SAG-M) which gives red cells a shelf life of 30–35 days. These are generally used for patients with anaemia requiring red cell transfusion.
• All red cells for transfusion in the UK have been passed through a leucocyte depletion filter to reduce reactions to leucocytes in patients sensitized to human leucocyte antigens (HLA) (e.g. multiply transfused patients), to reduce incidence of sensitization to HLA antigens and to reduce risk of transmission of CMV. Leucodepletion reduces the theoretical risk of transmission of new variant Creutzfeldt–Jacob disease (nvCJD; see Chapter 49).

Directed donations, e.g. within families, are not considered ethical within the UK. Salvage of autologous blood which is then washed and transfused may be carried out during major surgery, e.g. liver transplantation.

Platelet transfusion

A single donor unit is prepared from a unit of whole blood by centrifugation within hours of collection. It contains approximately 5×10^{10} platelets in 50–60 mL fresh plasma; shelf life of 4–6 days. The standard adult dose is five pooled units group ABO and Rh compatible, but not cross-matched. Patients sensitized to HLA antigens may require platelets from HLA-compatible donors. Platelet transfusions are not generally used in patients with accelerated platelet destruction, e.g. immune thrombocytopenic purpura (ITP; see Chapter 41).

Indications

• Thrombocytopenia <50 × 10^9/L – in the presence of significant bleeding or prior to an invasive procedure.
• Thrombocytopenia <10 × 10^9/L or higher in patients with infection or bleeding. Prophylactic platelet transfusions are required in patients post-chemotherapy or stem cell transplant or with marrow failure or in patients with severe thrombocytopenia who are to have red cell transfusions.
• Platelet function defects (in presence of bleeding or prior to surgery), disseminated intravascular coagulation (DIC; see Chapter 43) and dilutional thrombocytopenia following massive transfusion.

Drugs that stimulate platelet production by binding with the thrombopoietin receptor-cMpl on progenitor cells and megakaryocytes, e.g. eltrombopag or romiplostim, are reducing requirements for platelet transfusions.

49.1 Complications of transfusion of blood components

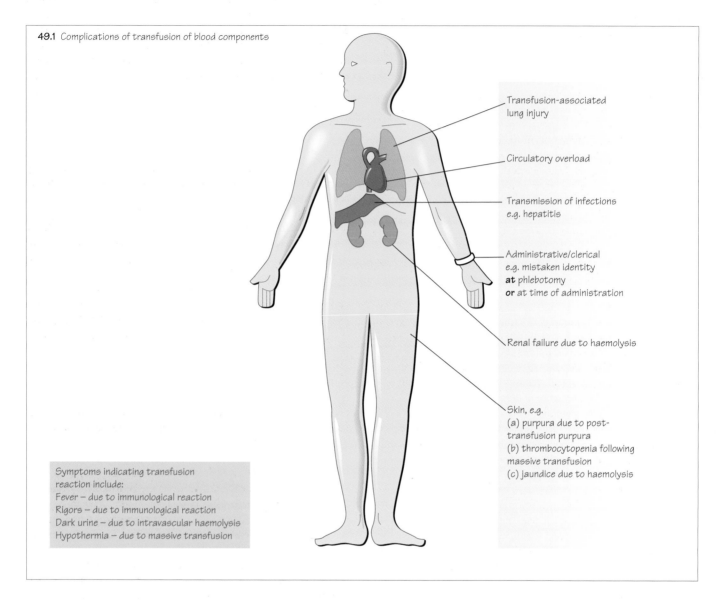

Transfusion-associated lung injury

Circulatory overload

Transmission of infections e.g. hepatitis

Administrative/clerical e.g. mistaken identity **at** phlebotomy **or** at time of administration

Renal failure due to haemolysis

Skin, e.g.
(a) purpura due to post-transfusion purpura
(b) thrombocytopenia following massive transfusion
(c) jaundice due to haemolysis

Symptoms indicating transfusion reaction include:
Fever – due to immunological reaction
Rigors – due to immunological reaction
Dark urine – due to intravascular haemolysis
Hypothermia – due to massive transfusion

Fresh frozen plasma

Fresh frozen plasma (FFP) is a source of all coagulation and other plasma proteins. Compatibility testing is not required, but blood group compatible units are used. FFP from group AB donors may be used if the recipient blood group is unknown. As FFP is not heat sterilized and may transmit infection, solvent-treated FFP is safer in this regard.

Indications

- Coagulation factor replacement. Perform coagulation tests and platelet count prior to use. Patients with disseminated intravascular coagulation (DIC) or massive transfusion at risk of bleeding and with coagulation abnormalities may benefit. Single-factor deficiencies are best treated with a specific factor concentrate.
- Liver disease – in the presence of bleeding or prior to invasive procedures, e.g. liver biopsy; combined with vitamin K.
- Haemolytic uraemic syndrome or thrombotic thrombocytopenic purpura usually with plasma exchange. Cryoprecipitate-poor FFP is preferred.
- Reversal of warfarin or direct factor Xa or factor II inhibitor anticoagulation or thrombolytic therapy.

Cryoprecipitate

Cryoprecipitate is prepared from the precipitate formed from FFP during controlled thawing, resuspended in 20-mL plasma. It is rich in fibrinogen, fibronectin and factor VIII. Group compatible units are used. It may be useful in patients with DIC, liver disease, following massive transfusion and, rarely, in von Willebrand disease.

Other blood products

These are derived from pooled human plasma that has undergone a manufacturing process designed to concentrate and sterilize the component. They carry a theoretical risk of transmitting diseases caused by prions (e.g. nvCJD). There have been no fully documented cases of this with blood products other than red cell transfusions, but the current UK practice is to use products made by recombinant DNA or plasma from non-UK donors.

Coagulation factor concentrates

Coagulation factor concentrates are available as freeze-dried powder of high purity. Factor VIII concentrate is used for treatment of haemophilia A and von Willebrand disease; recombinant factor VIII is now available. Factor IX concentrate, also available as recombinant, is used in patients with haemophilia B. Factor IX complex (prothrombin complex) also contains factors II, VII and X and is of value in patients with specific disorders involving factors II and X, oral anticoagulant overdose, in severe liver failure and to overcome inhibitors to factor VIII in patients with haemophilia A who have developed inhibitors. Its use carries a risk of provoking thrombosis and DIC.

Other concentrates include protein C, antithrombin, factors VII, XI and XIII. They are used in the corresponding congenital deficiencies. Protein C concentrate is also used in severe DIC, e.g. meningococcal septicaemia.

Recombinant human factor VIIa

This may be used for patients with massive uncontrollable haemorrhage post-trauma and surgery. It may cause thrombosis. It is extremely expensive.

Albumin solution

Albumin solution is available as 5%, 20% and 20% salt-poor formulations. It contains no coagulation factors. It is used in the treatment of hypovolaemia, particularly when caused by burns, and shock associated with multiple organ failure. Synthetic plasma volume expanders (e.g. dextrans, gelatin and hydroxyethyl starch) are of equal value in initial management. These 'colloids' remain longer within the intravascular space than 'crystalloid' solutions (e.g. 0.9% NaCl), exert a colloid osmotic effect and may elevate blood pressure. Resistant oedema in patients with renal and hepatic disease requires 20% albumin.

Immunoglobulins

Immunoglobulins (Igs) are prepared from pooled donor plasma by fractionation and sterile filtration. Specific Igs include hepatitis B and herpes zoster, which provide passive immune protection. Standard human Ig for intramuscular injection is used for prophylaxis against hepatitis A, rubella and measles, whereas hyperimmune globulin is prepared from donors with high titres of the relevant antibodies for prophylaxis of tetanus, hepatitis A, diphtheria, rabies, mumps, measles, rubella, cytomegalovirus and *Pseudomonas* infections.

Intravenous Ig may be used especially in the winter to protect against infections in patients with congenital or acquired immune deficiency. Infusions are given every 3–4 weeks. In high doses it is of value in some autoimmune disorders, e.g. immune thrombocytopenic purpura, Guillain–Barré syndrome.

White cell transfusion

White cell (buffy coat) transfusions prepared from normal donors or patients with chronic myeloid leukaemia have been used in neutropenic patients with life-threatening infection. There are few data demonstrating clinical efficacy.

Complications of transfusion (Fig. 49.1)

- **Administrative and clerical errors** must be avoided by rigorous adherence to procedures for checking and documentation when ordering, prescribing, issuing and administering blood components. These are by far the most common cause of serious and 'near miss' incidents.
- **Congestive heart failure** caused by circulatory overload.
- **Immunological reactions** may occur with transfusion of cellular and plasma-derived blood components. Haemolytic reactions are divided with 'acute' or 'delayed'. Acute reactions are due to preformed antibodies (e.g. anti-A or anti-B) usually IgM or complement fixing IgG, usually intraveascular and can cause fever, rigors, shock, DIC and acute renal failure. Delayed reactions occur after 3–10 days, usually due to IgG antibodies (e.g. Anti-Rh) and are extravascular (Table 49.1). They typically present with anaemia, jaundice, splenomegaly and fever.

Hypersensitivity reactions to plasma components may cause urticaria, wheezing, facial oedema and pyrexia but can cause anaphylactic shock, especially in IgA-deficient subjects. The transfusion must be stopped immediately. For severe reactions, the clerical details must be checked and samples from the donor unit and recipient are analysed for compatibility and haemolysis. Recipient serum is analysed for presence of atypical red cell, leucocyte, human leucocyte antigen (HLA) and plasma protein antibodies. Support care to maintain blood pressure and renal function and to promote diuresis and treat shock

Table 49.1 Haemolytic transfusion reactions

	Immediate	Delayed
Timing	Within 1 hour	7–10 days
Antibody	IgM (e.g. anti-A, anti-B)	IgG (e.g. anti-RhD)
Clinical	Headache, backache, hypotension	Nil or mild fever, 'jaundice'
	Renal failure	
Laboratory	Haemoglobinaemia	Raised bilirubin ± anaemia
	Haemoglobulinaemia	
	Methaemalbuinaemia	
Mortality	5–10%	0–1%

(intravenous steroids, antihistamines, adrenaline in severe cases) may be necessary.

• **Transmission of infection.** *Bacterial infections* can occur through failure of sterile technique at the time of collection or because of bacteraemia in the donor. *Protozoal infections* (e.g. malaria) can be transmitted and at-risk donors are not eligible to donate. *Viral infection* can be transmitted in spite of mandatory screening, as seroconversion may not have occurred in an infected donor, the virus may not have been identified or the most sensitive serological tests may not be routinely performed (e.g. testing for antihepatitis B core antibodies). The risk of transmission is much lower for those blood products that have undergone a manufacturing and sterilization process. There are a few documented cases of transmission of nvCJD by red cell transfusions.

• **Other complications.** Iron overload occurs in multiply transfused patients with refractory anaemia (see Chapter 10). Graft versus host disease may be caused by transfusion of viable T lymphocytes into severely immunosuppressed hosts, so cellular components should be irradiated prior to transfusion to fetuses, premature neonates, stem cell transplantation recipients, patients who have received fludarabine, patients with Hodgkin lymphoma and other severely immunocompromised patients.

Appendix: cluster of differentiation nomenclature system

Cell surface markers are molecules in the cell membrane that can be recognized by reactivity with specific monoclonal antibodies. Their presence gives information about the lineage, function or stage of development of a particular cell population. The cluster of differentiation (CD) nomenclature system groups together antibodies recognizing the same surface molecule (antigen).

T-cell markers	Remarks
CD number	
1a, b, c	Thymocytes, Langerhans' cells (CD1a)
2	E-rosette receptor. All T cells
3	T-cell receptor. Mature T cells
4	T helper/inducer subset
5	T cells (aberrantly expressed in B-CLL, mantle cell lymphoma)
7	T cells (aberrantly expressed in some AML)
8	T cytotoxic/suppressor
B-cell markers	
CD number	
19	B cells, including early B cells
20	Mature B cells
21	Mature B cells. C3d receptor, EBV receptor
22	B cells
23	Activated B cells
38	Plasma cell
79	B-cell antigen receptor
103	Hairy cells
138	Plasma cells
Myeloid and other markers	
Myeloid markers	
CD number	
11a, 11b, 11c	Adhesion molecule ligand. Also expressed on some B and T cells and monocytes
13	All mature myeloid cells
33	Myelin-associated protein. Early myeloid cells
61	Early myeloid cells
117	Early myeloid cells
Others	
CD number	
14	Monocytes, macrophages
25	IL-2 receptor-activated B cells
34	Stem cells
45	Leucocyte common antigen: all haemopoietic cells
56	Natural killer cells
9, 29, 31, 41, 42	Platelet markers
71	Red cell precursors
TdT	Terminal deoxynucleotidyl transferase – early B- and T-cell precursors

Index